UNDERSTANDING EEG

UNDERSTANDING EEG

An Introduction to Electroencephalography

Donald Scott

J. B. Lippincott Company
Philadelphia

First published in 1976 by
Gerald Duckworth & Co. Ltd.
The Old Piano Factory
43 Gloucester Crescent, London NW1
Distributed in the United States by
J.B. Lippincott Company, Philadelphia, Pa.

ISBN 0 397 58188 2
Library of Congress Catalog Card No. 75 39289

Typeset by John Swain (Glasgow) Ltd.
Printed by Unwin Brothers Limited, Old Woking

By the same author

Neurological and Neurosurgical Nursing (Pergamon) 1966

About Epilepsy (Duckworth) 1969 (2nd ed. 1973)

The Psychology of Work (Duckworth) 1970

Fire and Fire Raisers (Duckworth) 1974

Contents

Preface

The existence of electrical potentials originating from the human brain, recordable on the scalp – the EEG – is a relatively recent discovery, only 45 years old. As a result, advances continue not only in technology but also in the value of findings in clinical practice. Currently the procedure has a particular place in the investigations of patients with neurological problems and a variety of other disorders which affect the nervous system. However, the electroencephalographer has made perhaps too little effort to explain the difficulties of the techniques that he employs and his findings to the 'users'. For this reason patients are often referred inappropriately and the reports furnished are misunderstood, leading to a poor reputation for electroencephalography in the eyes of many clinicians. I regard this reputation as unjustified, and in fact this book is an attempt to redress the balance, to improve communications, to indicate what the electroencephalographer feels and what advances can be expected in the field in the near future.

The aim of the book is to explain simply what an EEG is, what diagnostic information it can provide and, as a corollary, what deductions cannot be made. I have written it for the senior medical student encountering EEG for the first time and for a variety of post-graduates studying for higher qualifications, for example Memberships of the Royal College of Physicians and the Royal College of Psychiatrists as well as Fellowships of Anaesthesia and Surgery. In addition general practitioners and others who receive reports from hospitals which include EEG information may find the book useful. Other groups who will, I hope, refer to it include nurses working in intensive therapy units, psychologists engaged in clinical and research work and a variety of people employed in the hospital, technical and scientific services.

The book arose from my wide experience of teaching and discussion with a whole range of people interested in brain activity and its significance, particularly undergraduates. The points they raised have gone a long way to shaping the account of EEG I put forward here. It derives from work carried out in a busy teaching hospital department where the diversity of clinical problems presented is almost infinite and research is constantly in progress. I have relied heavily on my colleagues and the investigations that we have undertaken together over the years in the department.

I have adopted a simple and forthright approach to the subject, removing as far as possible any mysteries that surround it. I have concentrated on general principles and have discussed topics under clinical headings rather than according to the EEG phenomena seen. I have not aimed to cover the field encyclopaedically. For example I have not included the EEG changes in every single condition, nor details of animal studies, except where essential for the understanding of a particular point. However, I feel the groundwork covered should form an adequate basis for those who wish to pursue the subject further. For this reason I have provided not only a list of texts for further reading but also a bibliography. To keep this to a manageable size I have concentrated largely on recent key references that are readily available. The bibliography serves as an entry point for the literature rather than a comprehensive reference list.

Although this is a brief text I have shown in various sections the importance of the appropriate methodological approach as well as techniques of quantification by visual means, areas which have not been as rigorously explored as they might have been and which in any case are not generally known to many clinicians. In addition recent advances and future developments have been discussed. It may be that my views will not be appreciated by all my colleagues who are specialists in the field, but I feel that there is a need for a book directed to the audience that I have indicated. No such volume exists in English, though excellent more detailed accounts of every aspect are available.

There is one further point that I should make. This is a book on electroencephalography. Nowadays many departments that carry out EEGs have the title 'Clinical Neurophysiology,' and they are engaged in a variety of studies assessing the peripheral as well as the central nervous system. I have devoted myself to the investigation of the central nervous system and therefore probably deserve the disparaging title given to me by a late colleague: 'You are the youngest old-fashioned consultant in clinical neurophysiology.' With these reservations I hope my comments, though not a final statement, will serve as a useful progress report on a discipline which is less than 50 years old.

Writing a book like this means necessarily relying on colleagues who have taught one and whose articles and books on the subject have been quoted. They are too numerous to name but I must mention the late James Margerison who helped me so much in getting to grips with EEG and with the problems it presents. Many of his provocative statements have unfortunately not been written down but they have provided a valuable stimulus to me, and in fact many of his comments figure in this book. I hope he would have approved. I am of course grateful to all those who have worked in my department over the years. I must mention especially Dr Pamela Prior who has contributed to so many studies, especially those on cerebral anoxia and in relation to the EEG computer file. In this context I must also acknowledge Mr B. Abbot and Miss D. Gillon of the London Hospital Computer Department for their help over the years. In addition I wish to thank Mr Douglas Maynard who has contributed in many areas, both in computer analysis of the EEG and the development of various new devices. Miss Sue Virden and other technicians in the department have given invaluable support. Dr Prior and Miss Virden have also been helpful in selecting material for illustrations. My warm thanks are expressed to Mrs Jean Held for her indefatigable secretarial help with various drafts, not only of this book but also of so many of our papers. I am also grateful to Mrs S. Richardson for typing most of the final manuscript. A word of appreciation must also got to the staff of my publishers who over the years have assisted me with various books, including this one, helping me to reach as high a standard of production as is possible.

Finally I am most grateful to my wife who has been a constant source of encouragement, and without whose help I should never have completed the work on this book.

D.F.S. 1975

CHAPTER ONE

What Happens in the EEG Department?

Electroencephalography (EEG) is the study of the small, constantly changing electrical potentials from the brain which can be recorded from the scalp. The technique was first described in man by a German psychiatrist, Berger, in 1929 (Gloor 1969), and although experience has been gained in this technique over the past forty-five years in relation to clinical medicine, many misconceptions abound, both about what is actually done in an EEG department and about what the recordings mean. It is a field which has come in for strong criticism from, for example, Matthews (1973) and Pappworth (1974). Some of these criticisms relate to the basic problems of recording and others to the subjective visual assessment of complex tracings. Further problems arise in the interpretation of what the findings imply for particular diagnoses. The clinician does not always understand which particular patient would be a suitable referral or the terms used in the EEG report. The EEG, in itself, is a painless and non-invasive procedure although from the technical point of view it is complex.

The EEG is nowadays used by doctors in nearly every hospital ward and department (Table 1.1). The neurologist employs it as an aid to diagnosis and assessment particularly in patients with epilepsy. The neurosurgeon makes use of it

Table 1.1 Source and age distribution of EEG referrals

(a) Source of EEG referrals		*(b) Age distribution of EEG referrals*	
Neurological	30%	0–1 years	4%
General medical	20%	2–5 years	5%
Cardiac and Intensive Care	13%	6–15 years	12%
Neurosurgical	12%	16–69 years	73%
Pediatric	12%	70 and over	5%
Psychiatric	5%		
Other	8%		

as a means of investigation of patients with possible brain tumours. The general physician finds prognostic help in it with unconscious patients after cardiac arrest, and it can be a sensitive indicator of impending hepatic encephalopathy in patients with liver disease. The psychiatrist employs it for patients in whom he believes there is an organic basis for a mental disorder, for example those with pre-senile dementias. The paediatrician concerned with the various forms of childhood epilepsy refers patients for it, as do those concerned with neonatal brain damage. The general surgeon has recourse to it in patients who have collapsed during or after operation or those who have suffered head injuries. The ENT surgeon finds that, with increasing sophistication of the apparatus, disturbance of 8th cranial nerve function can now be investigated using special EEG techniques. There is also a wide variety of research uses for EEG in neuropharmacology and psychology.

Because some of the difficulties of the EEG relate simply to the fact that a mystery attaches to what is done in the EEG department, I propose in the first chapter to 'lift the veil' explaining in simple terms the techniques of the examination. As the book continues, the significance of the various findings will emerge and what they mean will be explained.

The EEG request form

The EEG request form is the main channel of information between the referring doctor and the electroencephalographer, who is almost invariably medically qualified. The recordings are carried out by EEG technicians who, although not doctors, have their own special course of training and examination as well as career structure. The EEG request appears complicated. This is not merely for its own sake, but to draw attention to the practical points which must be known before deciding whether the recording should be carried out in the department or at the bedside, as well as to establish vital information which will influence the conduct of the examination and the interpretation of the EEG – for example, information on the drugs the patient is taking.

This is a permanent record: please complete legibly and tick appropriate boxes: ☑

THE LONDON HOSPITAL, E.1.
Department of Neurology

REQUEST FOR ELECTROENCEPHALOGRAM (E.E.G.)

Remarks:
(eg.: urgent; portable; monitoring, etc.)
Date next O.P. Appt.

SURNAME | **First name** | **Mr. ☐ Mrs. ☐ Miss ☐** | **AGE** | **HOSPITAL RECORD NO.**

ADDRESS IF O.P. | **Hospital if not L.H.**

CONSULTANT/ referring doctor / | **O.P./Ward** | **AMBULANT ☐ CHAIR ☐ BED ☐**

REASON FOR EEG | **FOCAL BRAIN LESION SUSPECTED ?** ☐ | **WHERE**

SUMMARY OF HISTORY AND EXAMINATION
If fits occur state type, frequency, F.H., etc.:

HISTORY: Head injury ☐ Craniotomy ☐ ECT ☐ leucotomy ☐ 1° Neoplasm ☐

STATE: Drowsy ☐ Stupor ☐ Coma ☐ Disturbed ☐

DIAGNOSIS

RESULTS OF INVESTIGATIONS
e.g. neuroradiology etc.

METABOLIC ABNORMALITY: Uraemia ☐ B12 ☐ Glucose ☐ Hormone ☐ Calcium ☐ Other ☐

MEDICATION (not to be stopped for EEG)
relevant details of present therapy:

ANTICONVULSANT ☐ SEDATIVE ☐
PSYCHOTROPIC ☐ OTHER ☐
HORMONE ☐ NONE ☐

Previous EEGs elsewhere | **DATE**

EEG REPORT | **EEG No.:**
Date:

Figure 1.1 The EEG request form as used at the London Hospital

These and many other points are needed, and some of these are shown on the request form illustrated (Fig. 1.1). On receipt of the request form, a priority is assigned, if this has not already been indicated by the referring clinician. This is necessary as there is of course a limit to the number of tracings that can be carried out on any particular day because of the usual limitations of staff and space which apply to other service specialities. One problem with the EEG is that it requires about three quarters of an hour, including time for preparation, running the tracing and removal of the electrodes. In addition, there are the usual 'housekeeping' aspects of any department, including checking apparatus and electrodes, as well as filing records, and arranging appointments.

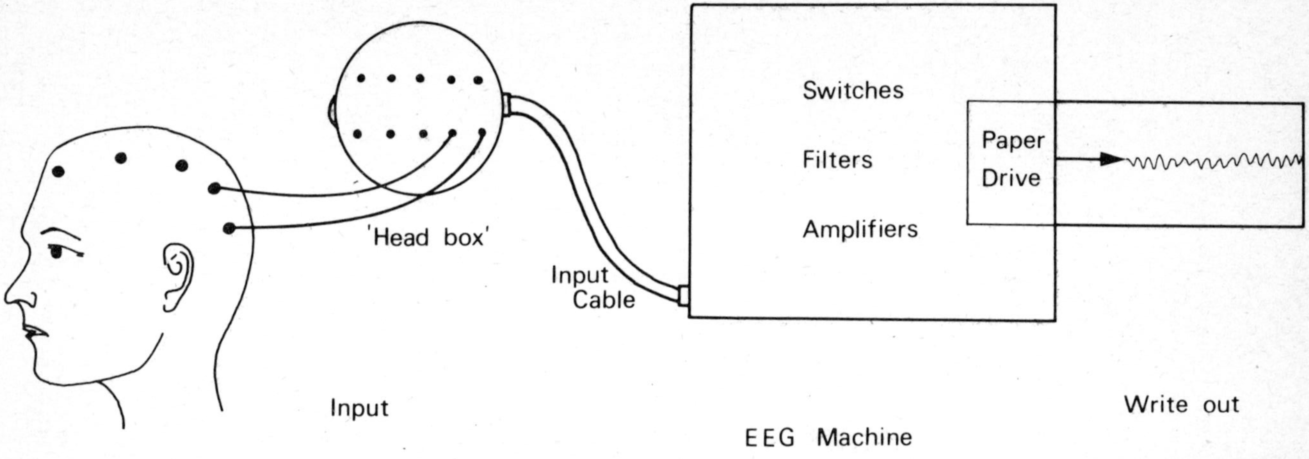

Figure 1.2 The basic system indicating the input, the machine itself and the write-out

The recording

The patient represents the main part of the 'input' end of the recording system, which has two other parts: the EEG machine proper and the third, the 'write-out' (Fig. 1.2). It is important that the patients should be prepared for the test, that is to say that he is aware that it will take a definite time to perform. Some patients are frightened that they are having 'shock treatment' – a fear built up in the minds of many from seeing the film *A Clockwork Orange*. For this and other reasons the technician's first job is to settle the patient, who generally is told to take usual meals and medicines before the test.

When appointments are sent to outpatients they are accompanied by a special letter explaining the test and pointing out in particular that the hair will have to be disturbed to get the electrodes in place, so that it is better not to have a special coiffure on the day of the recording. Lacquer and other hair dressings should be avoided since they also impede the process of preparation and can sometimes cause poor contact between scalp and the electrodes. A relaxed patient makes for a recording free of muscle artefact which, as will be seen later, may mar the EEG tracings and completely obscure the relevant brain potentials.

Electrode placement

The electrodes, at least 19 in all, are placed on the scalp according to a standard plan. The plan most commonly used is that put forward by an International Committee in 1958 (Jasper 1958). The positions of the electrodes are determined by measurement from landmarks on the skull, namely the inion, the nasion and the mastoid processes. The measurements have to be proportional to the skull size and shape, and so that the system is applicable to children as well as to adults. The electrodes are designated by letters and numbers. The letters indicate the area of the brain underneath the electrode: for example, F for frontal, P for parietal, etc. The odd numbers denote those on the left side of the head and the even ones those on the right (Fig. 1.3). Hence P4 is the

Key to electrode 'Names'

Fpl	—	Left fronto-polar
Fp2	—	Right fronto-polar
F3	—	Left superior frontal
F4	—	Right superior frontal
F7	—	Left inferior frontal/anterior temporal
F8	—	Right anterior temporal/inferior frontal
Fz	—	Mid frontal
C3	—	Left central or rolandic
C4	—	Right central or rolandic
Cz	—	Vertex
T3	—	Left mid temporal
T4	—	Right mid temporal
T5	—	Left posterior temporal
T6	—	Right posterior temporal
P3	—	Left parietal
P4	—	Right parietal
Pz	—	Mid parietal
O1	—	Left occipital
O2	—	Right occipital

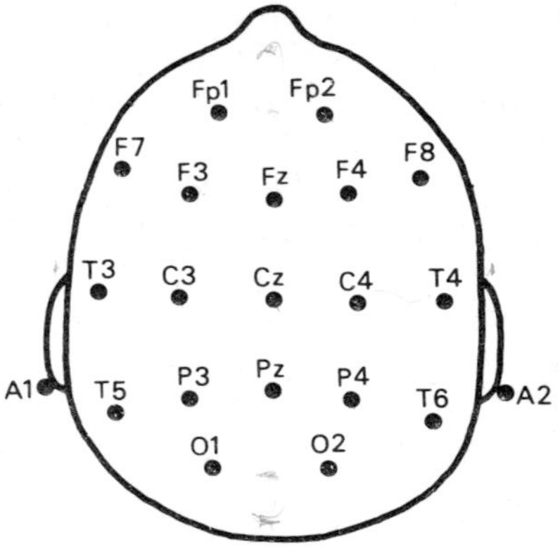

Figure 1.3 The 'head diagram' shows the electrode labelling according to the 10–20 system. The labelling of most electrodes is self-explanatory (odd numbers on the left side, even on the right). The mid-line electrodes are designated by z, for example, Fz, as they have a zero measurement from the mid-line

right parietal electrode. The system is called the 10/20 system because the distance between bony points, for example the inion and the nasion, is divided into lengths either 10% of 20% of the total distance between these points. Thus the frontal polar point is 10% up from the nasion and the frontal electrode is a further 20% along the same line (For details see Jasper 1958).

The positions of these electrodes relative to the underlying brain structures were determined in two different ways. In the first method metal clips were placed along the fissures at neurosurgical operations. Subsequently electrodes were attached to the scalp and X rays were then taken. They showed up the clips and allowed the relationships of the electrodes to these to be determined. The other technique was on cadavers. The electrodes were stuck in position and holes drilled through them and the skull. The underlying cortex was marked through the holes with Indian ink. The brain was then removed so that the position of the electrodes could be related directly to the cortical surface.

The technician obviously examines the scalp in detail during measurement before electrode placement, marking points with a 'skin pencil'. As a result, quite often she detects asymmetries of the skull or sees scars on the scalp which have previously escaped notice.

The types of electrodes used can be divided into two groups: those for routine and those for special purposes (Fig. 1.4). The former group comprises two main sorts, the pad and the stick-on electrode. There is discussion and disagreement between electroencephalographers as to which are the most satisfactory, but the former are quicker to apply. Both sorts are about 1 centimeter in diameter and are made of silver coated with silver chloride to improve the electrical qualities. Whichever type of electrode is used, the hair is first parted and the scalp cleansed with acetone to remove any grease or scales, to obtain good electrical contact between scalp and electrode. The pad electrode consists of a short silver rod at the end of which is a pad of cotton wool the size of a finger tip, covered in lint soaked in saline. This electrode has a plastic mount which is held in place on the head with a series of stout rubber slats. These are put over the head and tied firmly, but not tightly, under the chin. The electrodes are put under the rubber and thus stay in place. Generally these electrodes are easier and quicker for the technician to apply, and there is less cleaning necessary afterwards than with the other variety of routine electrodes. The stick-on electrode is a small silver cup with a hole in the middle and a flange round the edge. The flange and the surrounding area of scalp after cleansing are spread with collodion, which is dried by a jet of air. Whichever type of electrode is used, a jelly containing saline acts as the

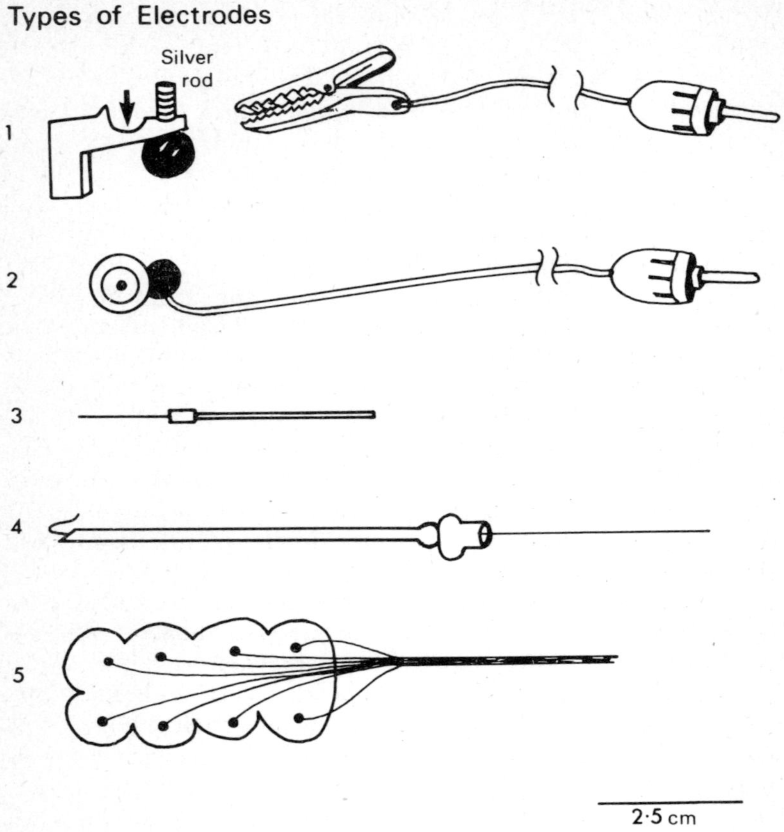

Figure 1.4 (1) The pad electrode with its plastic mount. The position of the rubber slat which holds it in place is indicated by the arrow. A crocodile clip is attached to the silver rod. This carries a lead with the plug which is inserted into the 'head box'
(2) The disc, stick-on electrode usually with a hole in the centre so that electrode jelly can be inserted. It has its own lead
(3) The sterilised needle electrodes which have their own lead and plug (not shown)
(4) The sphenoidal electrode. The needle is inserted and then withdrawn leaving the wire in place. This is insulated except at the tip.
(5) One type of corticography electrode – the 'plastic sheet' type. It is sterilised and placed in position by the neurosurgeon. The contact points are shown. The position on the cortex is maintained by surface tension.

conducting medium. It is rubbed on to the scalp before the pad electrode is put into place, or squirted into the cup of the stick-on electrode after this has been glued firmly to the scalp. The stick-on electrode is useful for restless patients and prolonged recordings. These electrodes can only be removed by acetone, which dissolves the collodion. It can then be combed from the hair at the end of the recording.

When all the electrodes are in place, they are connected to the EEG machine. Each stick-on electrode has a permanently attached lead, while pad electrodes are connected by a lead with a crocodile clip. These leads in both cases have a plug at the end, and this is inserted into the complex socket known as the 'head box' which in turn is attached to the EEG machine by a cable. The 'head box' has an individual socket which corresponds to each electrode on the head, so that the technician inserts the plugs systematically to link the patient to the apparatus.

Electrodes for special purposes include the small platinum needle electrodes suitable for quick insertion into the scalp of unconscious patients. These also have the advantage that they can be sterilised. Other special purpose electrodes include those for sphenoidal recordings, used in the assessment of patients with temporal lobe epilepsy, and those for electro-corticography, when recording is directly from the cortical surface. The techniques for this and their use will be described in Chapter 4.

The EEG machine

With the patient attached to the EEG machine we must consider this apparatus in outline. More details are provided by Cooper *et al.* (1974) and Kiloh *et al.* (1972), but essentially it is a device capable of amplifying the minute brain potentials measured in millionths of a volt and converting them into signals which can be displayed in various forms but generally as a permanent ink-on-paper record. However, the amplification system is only part of the contents of the apparatus. Because there are unwanted signals, such as high-frequency muscle activity and troublesome slow potentials, both high-frequency and low-

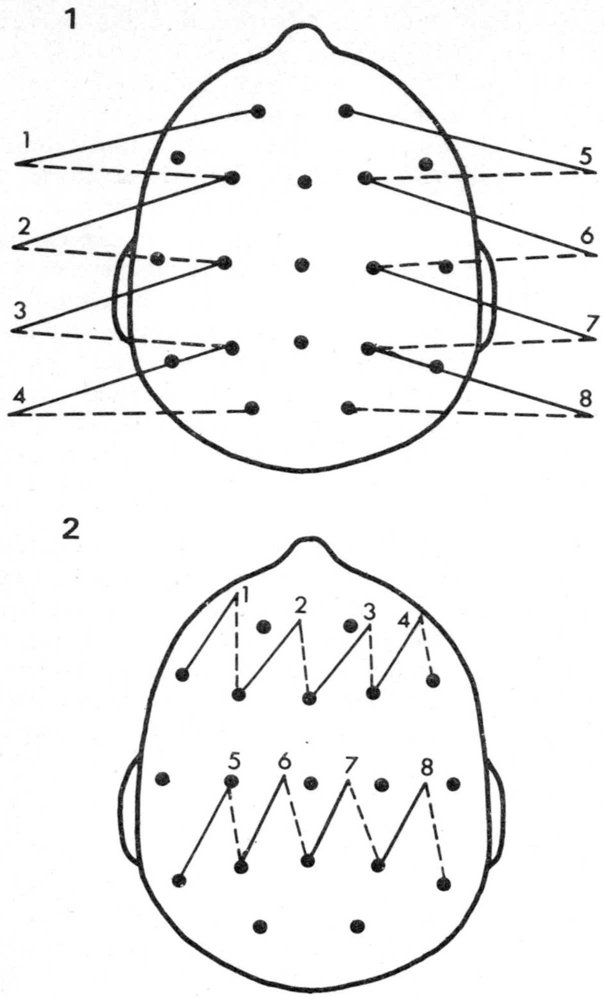

Figure 1.5 Two examples of the way in which electrodes are connected for recording. The electrodes connected to the 'black' leads are shown by solid lines. The numbers indicate which channel of the write-out will display the potentials from any particular pair of electrodes. (1) shows a parasagittal arrangement, (2) a transverse. Other types of arrangement are 'pre-set' so that the technician merely has to turn a knob to change the electrode connections

frequency filters are needed. In addition, the machine contains an elaborate series of switches, so that the electrodes can be linked in various ways to produce the EEG tracing. It is usual to have pre-set connections, so that at one stage of the recording the electrodes are connected in a longitudinal pattern from front to back, while later a transverse pattern of recording can be used (Fig. 1.5). The switching also has to allow for any special combinations which the technician may decide upon, as a result of observation of abnormality in the record. Part of her training consists in recognising abnormality; and often, depending on her skill at selecting types of electrode arrangement, interpretation of the EEG may be made not only simpler but also more accurate.

In order to record from a large proportion of the electrodes at any one time, the machine consists not just of one series of amplifiers and filters, but of 8, 12, 16 or more quite separate banks of these which operate separately. However, it is essential that each channel has the same characteristics. Thus one of the first things the EEG technician has to do before carrying out a record is to calibrate the machine to make sure that the amplification and sensitivity of each channel is the same. Then, if she makes alterations during the course of the tracing, it is her job to annotate it appropriately for the subsequent interpretations. The calibration is also carried out at the end of the EEG to make sure that no unrecognised faults have developed in the system during the course of the test (see Fig. 1.6).

The biological amplifier

Biological amplifiers used in EEG and for recording other physiological variables, such as ECG, are basically similar. There are two inputs to the amplifier, and the device is built in such a way that electrical signals, biological or external, affect each of the inputs in a similar fashion: the so called 'in-phase signals' are severely curtailed, whereas biological signals which are usually different, that is 'out of phase' are amplified. This ability of the biological amplifier to reject unwanted signals is known as 'discrimination', and a particular apparatus may have a discrimination ratio of 1 to

CMR — Common Mode Rejection

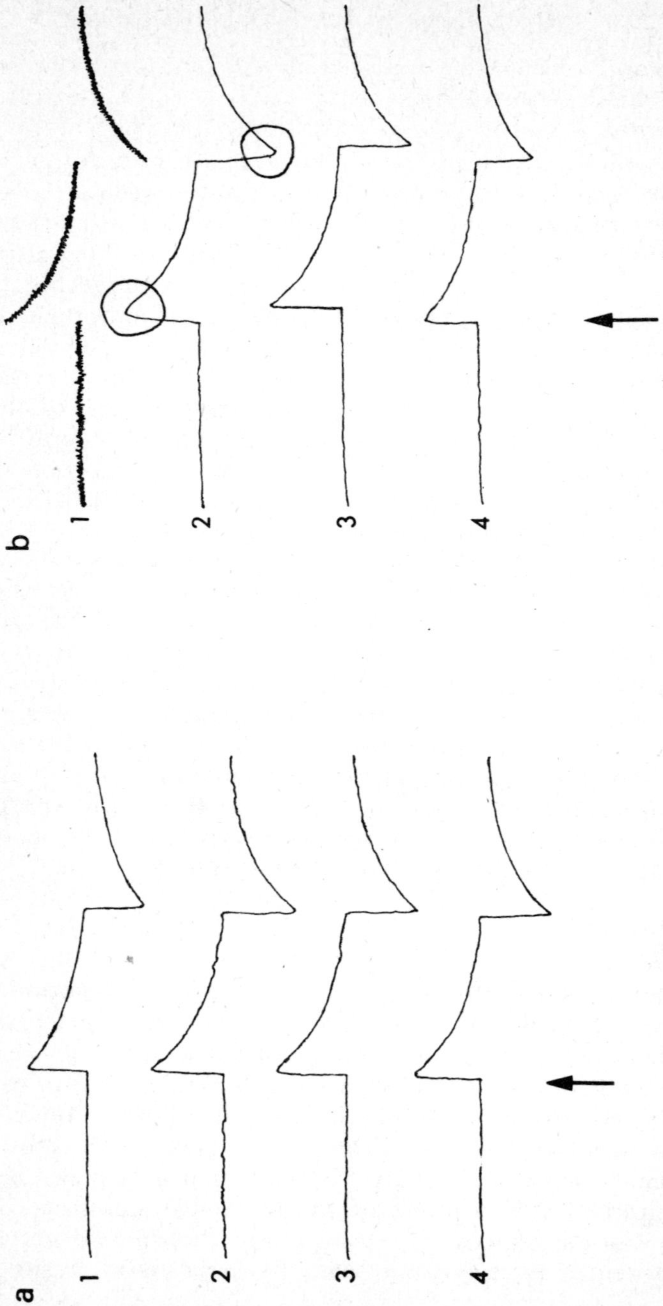
a
1
2
3
4
b
1
2
3
4

Figure 1.6 Calibration: Examples of the calibration procedure in two groups of four channels
(a) Each of the channels shows a similar size of deflection following the input of 50 microvolts into the system. The pens are all accurately lined up; the take off point is in line with the arrow indicated below. The tips of the deflections have the same 'pointedness' or degree of damping
(b) In contrast all four channels show a defect. (1) has excessive noise. (2) as indicated by the circles has a blunted tip — over damped. Channel (3) is out of alignment. Note that the take-off point is at least 2 millimetres further to the right than the other channels which are lined up with the arrow below. Channel (4) shows a deflection which is considerably smaller than the others, even though the input to that channel was also 50 microvolts

10,000. Such a feature is necessary since a variety of electro-magnetic radiations from electrical apparatus in hospitals may otherwise mask the tracings. Further problems of patient safety and isolation from the mains supply are also taken carefully into account in the design of EEG machines.

It is usual in physiological work to label the two inputs to an amplifier as the 'active' and the 'indifferent'. Both of course come from the individual under study: the former input from the source of the potential, the latter from an area presumed to be as near zero potential (see below) as is possible in a biological system. The difference between the outputs is amplified and appears on the 'write-out'. The direction of the deflection on the write-out depends on whether the potential applied to the active input is negative or positive. It is a convention of EEG for a negative potential to give rise to an upward movement of the pen (Fig. 1.7). This convention is absolutely fundamental to the understanding of EEG. As the convention also applies to each of the channels which has its own amplifying system and the same arrangement of inputs, the origin and distribution of cerebral potentials can be worked out by careful application of this convention and by varying types of electrode connections. We shall return to this point in Chapter 3 when these principles will be applied to a particular EEG disturbance.

There are two basic techniques for the recording. The first is the monopolar or common reference system and the second is the bipolar system. Both are used because of the

Grid 1 neg to Grid 2, pen deflects ↓

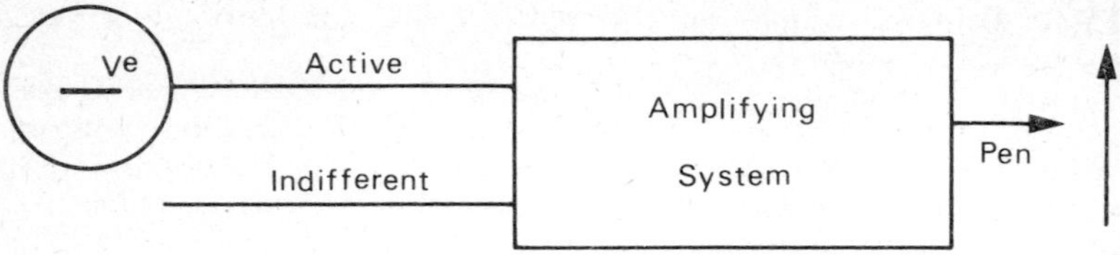

Figure 1.7 The EEG convention. The effect of a negative potential at the active input of an amplifying system leads to an upward deflection of the pen. The reverse is true if this potential affects the indifferent electrode and positive potentials have exactly equal and opposite effects

basic difficulty of finding an area of near-zero potential. The monopolar system often employs the ear-lobe as a relatively neutral source, but unfortunately it may pick up discharges from the temporal areas. Another reference point is the nose, but it may be affected by cardiographic potentials. For these reasons a slightly different technique called 'common average reference' is sometimes used. It depends on the fact that the electrical potentials from the brain are relatively random and that at any one moment the algebraic sum from all the electrodes considered together is near zero; that is, as many electrodes are becoming positive as negative and two types of potentials are cancelling each other out. In this technique the active input for any channel is connected to a single scalp electrode and the indifferent input is the algebraic sum of the potentials arising from all the other electrodes taken together.

The bipolar recording system employs another approach. Here the two inputs to the amplifier are connected to active electrodes, and as with other systems the write-out is the difference between them. In fact the various recording techniques are complementary, each yielding a different kind of information. This is important in localisation of abnormality, as we shall see in later chapters, particularly Chapter 3.

The write-out system

The write-out system consists of two main parts: the actual writing instrument, and the paper drive. The broad strip of

EEG paper is driven through the machine at a constant rate by an electric motor. The speed can be varied by the pressing of a button, but in much routine work the paper emerges from the EEG machine at the rate of 3 centimetres per second. It then moves across the bench-like top of the apparatus, at which the technician sits annotating the tracing as it emerges. If a particularly prolonged recording is carried out, say an all night sleep tracing or monitoring during a long surgical operation, very much slower rates of a few millimetres per second may be employed. This means that the tracing is of a more manageable size. The routine recording, which is about 15 minutes of actual EEG, consists of 90 pages. Each page represents 10 seconds at the standard speed of 3 centimetres per second and is about a foot long; the total length is 30 yards. Imagine seven family cars parked bumper to bumper by the kerb and this gives the length of a routine EEG. Fortunately for the electroencephalographer the paper is folded and he does not need to crawl along the pavement with his eyes down to report the EEG!

In routine work EEG signals are displayed as an ink trace on paper. The commonest output system simply uses a pen. but a more sensitive method is the ink jet. This, like the pen arm, is deflected by the fluctuating electrical signal created by the amplified brain potentials. EEG signals can also be displayed visually on a cathode ray oscilloscope or converted into sound as in the currently fashionable 'alpha' machine (see Chapter 15). Alternatively, the brain potentials can be recorded on magnetic tape so that at a later date they can be processed by a computer. The tape can be run repeatedly and a series of different programmes used for the analysis.

The EEG technician

As electroencephalographers we are naturally dependent to a great extent on our technicians. It is they who get the patient relaxed, attach the electrodes accurately, and make sure that the contact between the scalp and the electrode is satisfactory. If it is not, the tracing may be uninterpretable. Further, the technician makes careful notes about the patient. Has he had a recent fit? Is he taking drugs? When did he have his last meal? These and many other factors may modify the EEG recording. It may also be that some time has elapsed between the request form being sent for an outpatient and the recording actually being performed, the patient's condition having changed in the meantime. The technician may have to use special types of electrode placement or connections to bring out particular abnormalities. Also, during the routine EEG recording, apart from getting the patient to open and shut his eyes, the technician has to carry out two other procedures – so-called 'activation' procedures because they may 'bring out' pathological changes. In the first, hyperventilation, the patient is asked to breath deeply and steadily for three minutes. The second is photic stimulation, for which a stroboscope is used; this bright flashing light is now familiar because it is used widely in discotheques and for some stage shows. The rate of flashing can be controlled by the turn of a knob. Both forms of 'activation' lead to physiological changes and in certain individuals to pathological features as well (see Chapter 2).

When the recording has been completed, the technician once again carries out a calibration procedure. The electrodes are removed, the patient's scalp is cleaned and the hair is combed back into place. The technician's work, however, is not complete, and she has to finish her annotation of the record before taking it to a member of the medical staff responsible for reporting. In many departments she also makes a detailed descriptive report of the EEG, although obviously she is not trained to give an opinion on its diagnostic value. However, she is of course able to indicate, for example, that there is an abnormality which is generalised or localised as well as some of the other features seen.

The EEG report

In the next chapter we shall describe the normal EEG tracing and how abnormalities arise. To complete the saga of what happens in the EEG department, suffice it to say that a report is made. This report is divided into separate parts. It may give information about the patient's behaviour in the department: for example, a description of a fit, if this occurred. Next follows a detailed description of the EEG. Finally, there is a general comment or opinion on the likely clinical correlate. (The EEG report will be considered in detail in Chapter 14.) The report is typed on the bottom of the request form as shown in Fig. 1.1, while a copy of both the clinical information and the report itself are kept in the department for record purposes.

CHAPTER TWO

The Normal and Abnormal EEG

The problem of artefact

Having presented in outline how the EEG tracing is produced, we must now examine in more detail what it actually looks like. Though the question whether it is normal or abnormal is ultimately the main consideration, for the moment let us concentrate on what the tracings show rather than what they mean.

The first glance at an EEG tracing (Fig. 2.1), as I have often noted when teaching undergraduates, causes a puzzled expression. When the question is asked 'What is the most impressive thing?' potentials of non-cerebral origin are invariably singled out. Almost every page of any EEG shows something of this type, which we call 'artefact'. The electroencephalographer is in the opposite situation to the archaeologist. The archaeologist is delighted when he finds artefacts on his dig; the electroencephalographer is disturbed or even angered by them, especially if they could have been minimised by the technician when she was actually carrying out the recording.

Artefacts (Fig. 2.2 and Table 2.1) can be divided into two main kinds: first, biological potentials, like those caused by eye blinking; and secondly, potentials arising from the electrodes, the leads or the EEG machine itself. This second type, of course, are more amenable to correction. The technician learns to recognise them and to put matters right. The biological potentials present a somewhat different problem. The basic difficulty is that the brain waves are minute and can be completely masked by the much larger biological potentials. This is the recurring problem in EEG work. Putting it in more general terms, we are looking for a 'signal' and trying by all means possible to eliminate 'noise'. We shall come back to this point several times in the course of this book, especially in relation to computer-assisted methods used to enhance the 'signal' and reduce or eliminate the 'noise' (see Chapter 13).

Now we must return to the 'eyeballing methods of EEG assessment'. The on-going activity seen in the adult is generally of 20 to 40 millionths of a volt (microvolts), while the eyeblink artefacts arise because there is a positive potential at the front of the eyeball with respect to the back, which is about a 100 millivolts, i.e. thousandths of a volt. Movement of the eyeball upwards as a blink occurs affects the electrodes at the front of the head and causes large deflections on the EEG. Other eye movements cause similar effects. Even the cardiograph, conducted from the chest, may readily be recordable with the scalp electrodes. When the list and illustrations are examined it will be seen just how many different types of artefactual potentials there are.

How then does the electroencephalographer succeed in reporting an EEG? Most important of all, he must be sceptical of everything he sees in the tracing. He considers the shape of a particular wave and its distribution. Shape is one of the main clues to the identification of artefactual potentials, as they are often large sudden deflections with a geometrical outline. Distribution is also important. For example, eye movement potentials occur over the front of the head, while those arising from the head-rolling movements on the pillow have the opposite kind of spread. Thus, by a combination of native wit and experience, it is usually possible to distinguish between artefactual and brain potentials. Just occasionally it is impossible, and further recordings must be done.

The normal EEG

'Alpha rythm' is the main activity seen in the EEG of the alert adult (see Fig. 2.3). It occurs at a frequency of 8 to 13 cycles per second and over the posterior parts of the head, usually in a symmetrical fashion. It may be slightly different on the two sides and this has been related to handedness, the alpha being of slightly augmented amplitude on the right side in right-handed subjects (Kiloh *et al.* 1972, Cabral and Scott

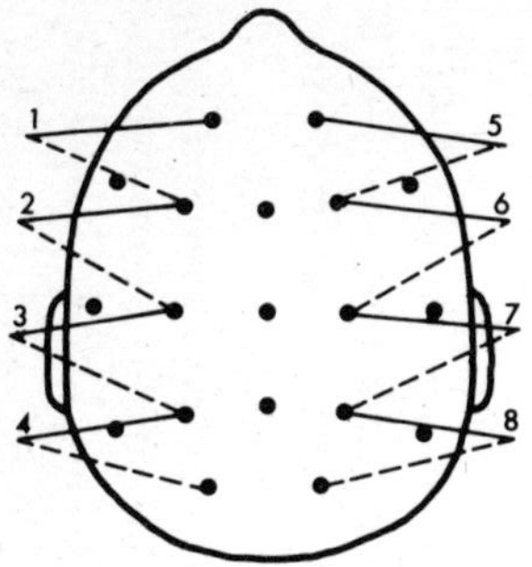

Control Settings

'gain' 50 µv

1 sec paper speed

High frequency filters HF 30 % above 70 Hz
Low frequency filters TC 0·3 sec

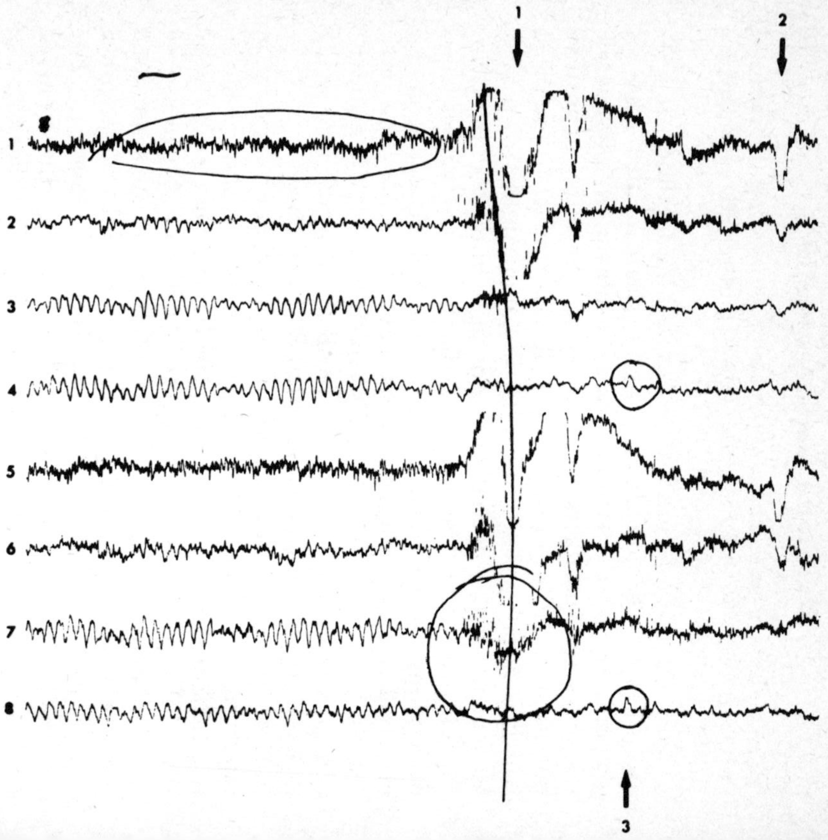

Figure 2.1 A typical example of a normal EEG recording. Note the artefacts indicated in channel 1: frontalis muscle potentials by the oval, eye opening artefact by Fig. '1', eye blink by Fig. '2'. The 11 cycle per sec alpha disappears when the eyes are opened, indicated by the line and the circle. Note at arrow 3 in channels 4 and 8 a small synchronous triangular deflection known as a 'lambda wave'. These appear when the eyes are open and moving over a patterned visual field. Note also the control settings indicating the amplitude of every given wave, 50 microvolts per centimetre; the speed of the recording, 3 centimetres per second; the high-frequency (HF) setting and the low-frequency setting, usually called a 'time constant' (TC). (The latter 2 are standard throughout, unless otherwise stated)

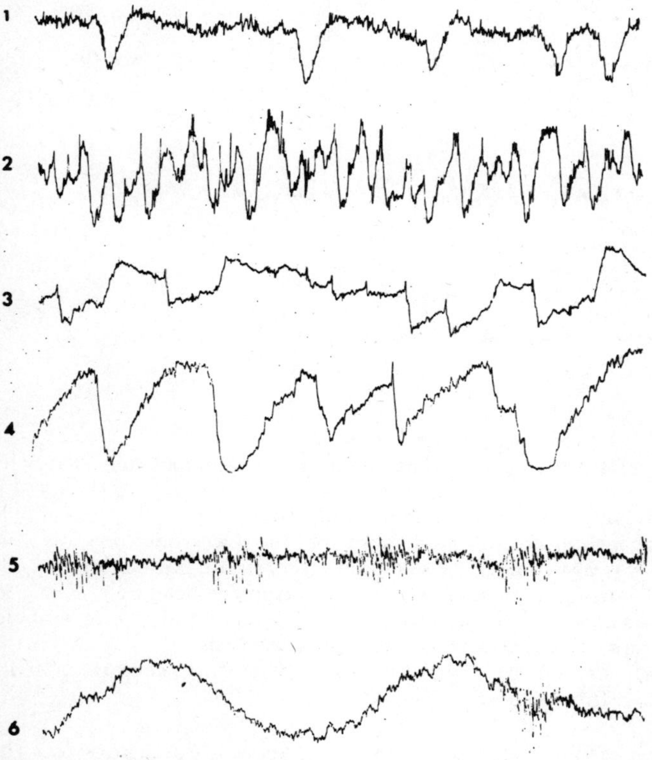

Figure 2.2 (a) Biological artefacts. (1) Eye blink. (2) Eyelid flutter. (3) and (4) Other eye movements. Note how (4) mimics delta activity. (5) Bursts of muscle spikes. (6) Sweat artefact.

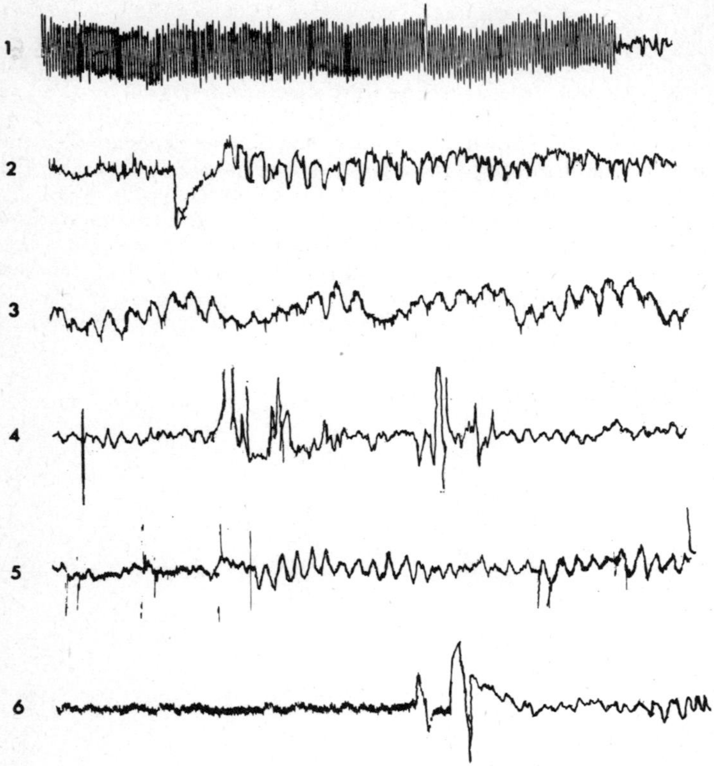

Figure 2.2 (b) Non-biological artefacts
1. Fifty-cycles artefact. Note that when it ceases some cerebral activity can be seen
2. Clip artefact. Note how it mimics sharp waves
3. Artefact produced by movement of the electrode, in this case because it was placed near the occipital artery – the pulse artefact
4. Artefact arising because of a faulty socket in the head box
5. 'Bleep' artefact. Note the grouped 'spikes' at the beginning and end of the section shown; these recur at regular intervals
6. Artefact created by 'dirty switch'. Note that cerebral activity returns when this has been corrected

1975). Opening the eyes leads to the disappearance of the alpha rhythm (Fig. 2.1) In the alert adult other types of activity appear. There is low-amplitude 'beta' activity with a frequency of over 13 cycles per second. It is usually

Table 2.1 Main types of artefact

(a) Biological – from the patient

1. Eyes	(a) Blinks – triangular deflections frontally
	(b) Movements – apparent slow waves fronto-temporally, varying depending on direction
	(c) Lid flutter – apparent frontal rhythmic activity repeated at 5–10 per second
2. Muscle	– Spikes usually in clusters, mainly in the temporal areas
3. 'Sweat'	– Very slow delta waves (lasting up to 4 seconds) frontally
4. ECG	– Usually the QRS complex, conducted from the heart (contrast pulse artefact) especially in common and average reference recording
5. Head and body movement	– Very variable in form and distribution, seen especially in children and unconscious patients (see Chapter 11)

(b) Non-biological – from the apparatus

1. Mains hum	– High frequency artefact (50 cycles per second in UK, 60 cycles per second in USA) arising from electrical apparatus, usually when contact between electrodes and scalp is poor
2. Electrode	– Due either to movement of electrode on the head or to electrode itself e.g. when near an artery (contrast cardiographic artefact), or arising from movement of the lead, many other causes, very variable wave form
3. 'Head box'	– Runs of rapid spikes caused by poor contact between electrode lead plug and socket
4. Switch and start-stop artefacts	– Sudden spike-like discharges, many due to 'dirty' switches; probably the most troublesome component in the EEG apparatus
5. 'Bleep' or telephone	– Regularly repeated artefacts caused by other hospital 'apparatus'

prominent in the frontal and rolandic regions and does not change with eye opening. 'Mu rhythm', runs of sharpened activity which has a comb-like appearance, may occur in the rolandic regions on both sides. This type of activity is a relatively infrequent finding and it does not change with eye opening. Interestingly enough, however, it does disappear when the subject is asked to move the arm or leg on the side opposite to the one on which the mu rhythm is occurring at that particular time. 'Lambda waves' (see Fig. 2.3) are seen

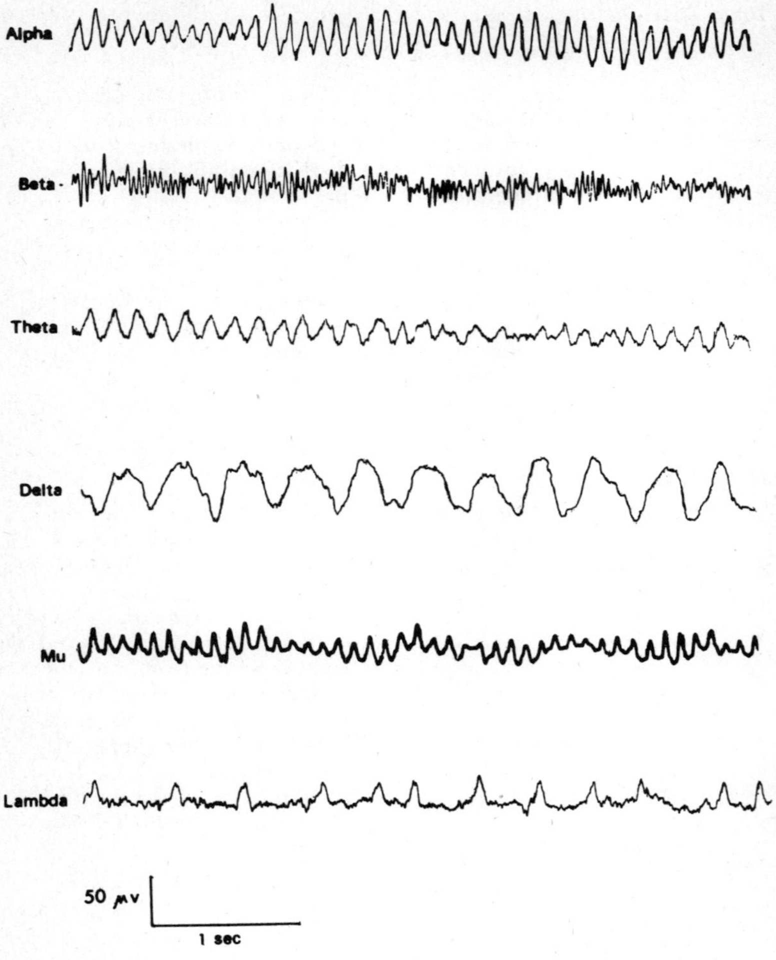

Figure 2.3 Normal activity seen in the EEG

over the occipital regions when the eyes are open and the subject is looking at a relatively complex pattern, for example at a picture. Often EEG departments are 'decorated' with travel posters, and these act as an excellent stimulus for the production of lambda waves. Each wave regularly follows an eye movement, and the amplitude depends on the level of the illumination and other characterists of the stimulus (Scott *et al.* 1969).

Three minutes of overbreathing is carried out during the routine EEG. This leads to a transient respiratory alkalosis in young adults and the appearance of episodes of symmetrical high-voltage frontal delta activity. These forms usually disappear within half a minute after overbreathing ceases. The response to overbreathing may be enhanced in hypoglycaemic subjects, in whom it may also be prolonged. Photic stimulation leads to triangular responses synchronously over both occipital regions related to the flash frequency.

'Theta' activity (see Fig. 2.3), which has a frequency range from 4 to below 8 cycles per second, and 'delta' activity with a frequency of less than 4 cycles per second are either scanty or absent in alert adults. In younger subjects episodes of theta may be seen frontally and also sharpened delta forms in the posterior temporal regions, with a slight right-sided preponderance. Both features are regarded as signs of an immature EEG, and these and other details of the maturation of brain activity will be considered later (see Chapter 8).

The EEG, and in particular the alpha rhythm, is influenced by many physiological as well as pathological disturbances of the body as a whole (Table 2.2). The amplitude and amount

Table 2.2 Physiological changes affecting the EEG

1. Age	Increase in frequency and many other changes (see Chapter 8)
2. Overbreathing	Produces episodic frontal delta activity in young adults
3. Drowsiness and sleep	Leads to a whole range of phenomena spindles, vertex sharp waves, lambdoid waves and K complexes
4. Diurnal/Nocturnal variation	Changes in alpha frequency occurring during the 24-hour cycle
5. Menstrual cycle	Alpha amount and frequency changes when the intermenstrual and premenstrual phases are compared (Margerison *et al.* 1964)
6. Hypoglycaemia	Leads to slowing of background activity with enhanced 'overbreathing' response
7. Hypothermia	Decreases amplitude of cerebral activity. At about 18 °C very little activity at all discernible
8. Hyperthermia	Increase in the amplitude of alpha frequency activity.

of alpha appear to vary independently, and sometimes these changes are too subtle to be quantified accurately by visual inspection alone. Frequency analysers, which split up the activity electronically into various frequency bands, can be employed (see Chapter 9). When this is done variation in the alpha rhythm is found at different phases of the menstrual cycle and even at different times of day (Harding 1971) if individuals are studied intensively. In EEG work, however, change in level of arousal is probably the most important and difficult thing to assess, and it may cause confusion when the electroencephalographer is determining the amount of abnormality (Scott *et al.* 1974).

Drowsiness and sleep

The earliest stages of drowsiness and light sleep are familiar. Imagine sitting in the train reading a newspaper; the paper momentarily goes out of focus and almost disappears. The train jolts over the points and the paper once more comes into focus. This sequence is repeated several times before sleep supervenes. The EEG in the earliest stages of sleep also shows a rapidly fluctuating pattern. Alpha momentarily increases in amplitude and rhythmicity, suddenly disappearing to leave a flattened trace characterised by a certain amount of low-voltage fast activity and some theta waves, corresponding to the stage when the newspaper was out of focus. Suddenly the alpha returns, only to disappear once more. After a spell in which the alpha thus waxes and wanes, sleep supervenes and the whole series of new phenomena appears.

Sleep phenomena (Fig. 2.4) are generally of high voltage and stand out clearly as background activity which is rather scanty, mainly low-voltage fast activity. There are 'vertex sharp waves', so called because they are prominent in that region and runs of 'sleep spindles'. These are components at 12 to 14 cycles per second, mainly frontally, and sometimes called 'sigma rhythm'. Triangular waves called 'lambdoid waves' appear in the occipital region at the same stage of sleep. As with most normal phenomena in the EEG in adults, all these components tend to occur at the same time, i.e.

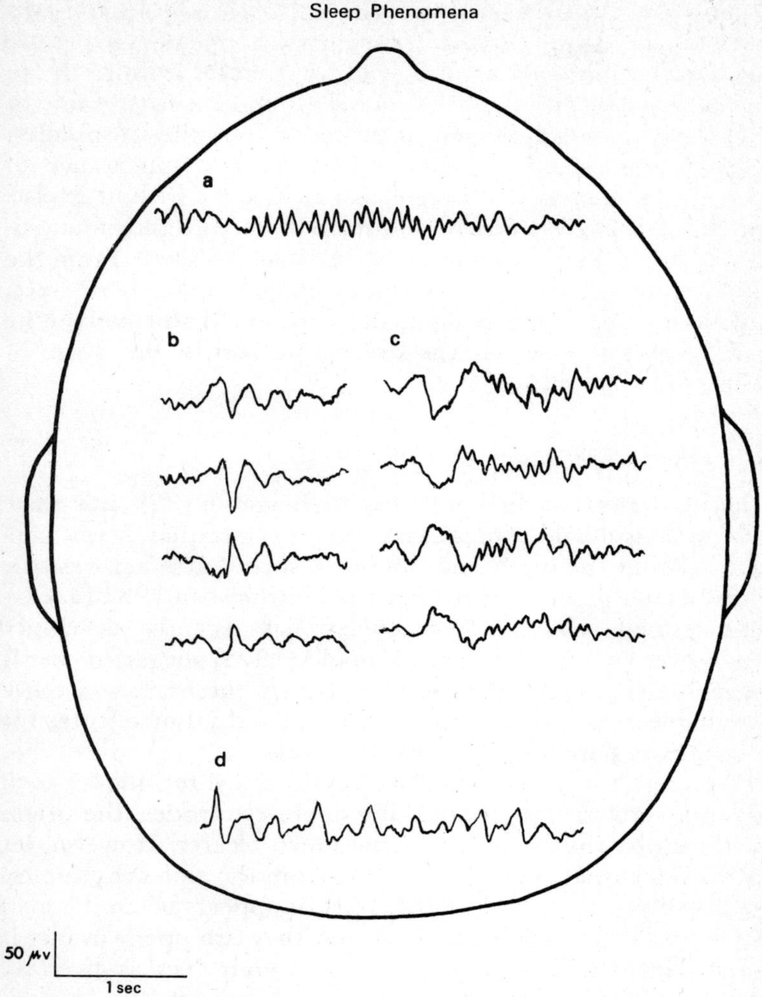

Figure 2.4 Sleep phenomena
(a) A run of sleep spindles which are usually prominent over the frontal regions
(b) An example of a vertex sharp wave and
(c) A K complex
Both (a) and (b) are prominent round the vertex although the latter usually has a much more widespread distribution
(d) Lambdoid waves which appear only over the occipital region

synchronously as well as of similar amplitude on the two sides. Deeper sleep is characterised by the appearance of delta activity. At this stage a noise or other stimulus leads to the so called 'K complex'. This is generalised and consists of one or more delta waves followed or preceded by trains of spindles. Even deeper sleep is characterised by the appearance of high-voltage generalised irregular delta activity with little else. Suddenly this gives way in undisturbed sleep to the paradoxical or Rapid Eye Movement (REM) stage of sleep. From the EEG point of view this is like a much more alert state, although the subject is difficult to rouse. If this is done he will be able to recount the dreams he had in this stage of sleep (see Chapter 10).

The origin of the alpha rhythm

The alpha rhythm, first described by Berger in 1929, was greeted by considerable scepticism; but the fact that is was genuinely from the brain and not some sort of artefact was confirmed by the work of Adrian and Matthews in 1934 (a & b). Interestingly enough, controversy has recently developed again over the alpha rhythm. Lippold (1973) suggested that it is generated by the eyes rather than by the brain – a quite untenable view, as a symmetrical alpha rhythm occurs, for example, in patients with only one eye!

As a result of advanced neurophysiological techniques such as intra-cerebral recording using micro-electrodes, the origin of the alpha rhythm is becoming much clearer. However, let us consider what we can determine from the alpha rhythm by observation of the scalp EEG. First, it appears when the eyes are shut and is usually absent when they are open. In fact it disappears when the command 'Open your eyes' is given by the technician rather than when the eyes are actually opened. This suggests that alerting blocks off alpha rhythm rather than visual stimulation, an observation confirmed by giving mental arithmetic to subjects with their eyes shut. Even the initial instructions abolish the alpha rhythm, and when, for example, 7 has been subtracted from 100 and the correct answer is given by the subject, his alpha again becomes quite prominent before the next problem is set. Hence, the alpha is blocked by mental activity and seems to be characteristic of the 'idling' state. Then presumably a large proportion of the cells are all behaving in a similar manner and the summed potentials on the scalp are seen as the alpha rhythm. When a problem is given to the subject, the cells take up their own, as it were, 'individual tasks' and produce activity at different frequencies, and the potential resulting as found by scalp recording is negligable. Another point of interest, obvious on inspection of scalp recordings when mental arithmetic is being performed, concerns the distribution of the diminution of the alpha. This is greater over the left hemisphere, which is known from other sources to be concerned with such tasks.

Secondly, the alpha rhythm is described as synchronous. This is not only because it is similar over the two hemispheres but because there is an exact temporal relationship between the two sides. Thus, if we consider an individual alpha wave appearing in the right parietal region, at the same time a similar wave will be appearing in the left parietal region. They will reach a peak and decline with identical timings. This strongly suggests that the alpha rhythm is controlled by a mid-line pace-maker. The alpha itself, we know, originates in the cerebral cortex, because in patients with unilateral lesions involving a local area of cortex the alpha is diminished or abolished in that region and is normal on the opposite side.

Having considered the origin of the alpha rhythm viewed from the scalp we must try to relate it to neural events. As the alpha rhythm generally has a frequency of 10 cycles per second the individual wave lasts 100 milliseconds. This contrasts strikingly with the duration of neural potentials as recorded by micro-electrode techniques; for example, the axonal action potentials last about half a milli-second. So it seems unlikely that they are responsible for the EEG. As a result of a great deal of research, it appears that the EEG is generated in the dendrites rather than the axons of the large cortical pyramidal cells which are uniformly oriented perpendicularly to the surface. These dendritic potentials are of the appropriate duration and amplitude and have been shown by simultaneous intracellular and surface recording techniques to correspond in timing. More details of this complex and as yet incomplete picture of the origin of brain rhythms are to be found in Andersen and Andersson (1968), McComus in Kiloh *et al.* (1972) Ellul (1973), Da Silver *et al.* (1973).

The reticular formation

The cerebral activity must now be considered in a wider context, not just the cortex and its mid-line connections, but more specifically the mid-line structures themselves. The thalamus is particularly important because it has been shown in animals that unilateral lesions lead to abolition of the on-going cortical activity on that side. The other mid-line region of significance is the reticular formation, as it is concerned not only with normal states such as sleep but pathological states like coma. It is a diffuse complex of nerve cells and fibres occupying the large central regions throughout the length of the brain stem and in continuity with the thalamic nuclei. There are widespread connections with cranial nerve nuclei, thalamic nuclei, the hypothalmus and the caudate nucleus. The reticular formation receives widespread sensory inputs from the whole body through connections with the posterior columns and the spinothalamic tracts. In addition, there are links with special sensory systems such as the eye and the ear.

Though the reticular formation as such was not discovered until much later, Bremer (1935) showed that consciousness could be disturbed and the EEG changed to show high-voltage rhythmic slow activity by transection of the brain stem. It was for Magoun and colleagues (Lindsley *et al.* 1950) to delineate more exactly how this came about and to show that stimulation of the reticular formation could lead to alerting and the abolition of the slow activity.

The abnormal EEG

We are now in a position to consider the abnormal EEG. There are three possible patho-physiological sites at which 'lesions' cause abnormality (Fig. 2.5): first in the cortex itself; secondly, in the cortico-mid-line connections; and thirdly in the mid-line structures, especially the reticular

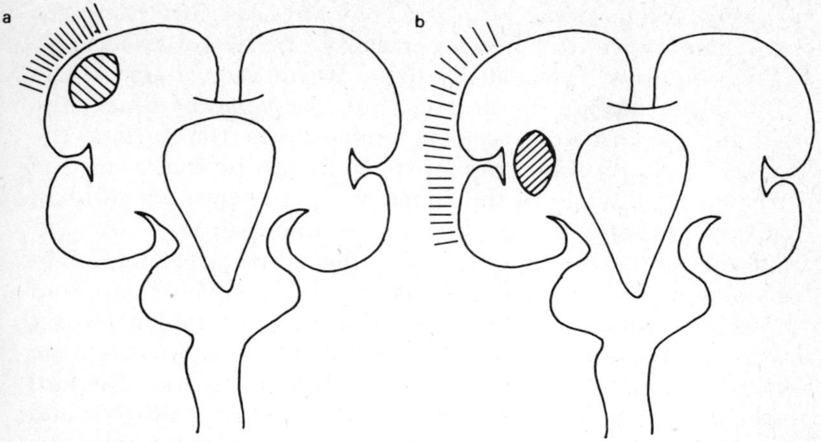

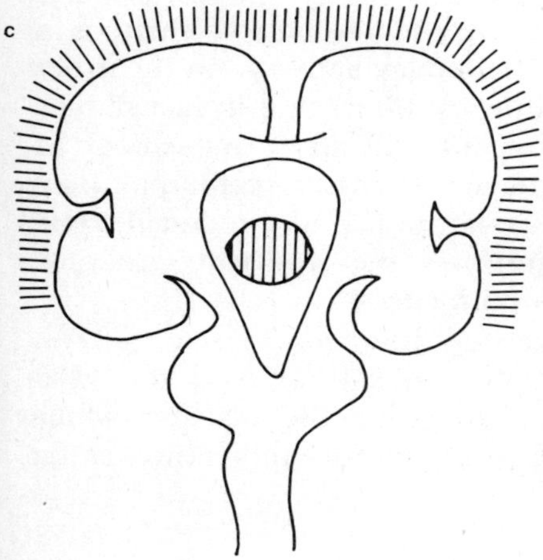

Figure 2.5 The lesions are shown with hatching, and any EEG abnormality by lines at right angles to the brain surface. In (a) the lesion is superficial and the EEG abnormality relatively localised. In (b) the lesion interrupts the pathways between the cortex and the mid-line structures, e.g. cortico-thalamic fibres, then the abnormality is more extensive than in (a) though still lateralised. (c) shows the effect of a mid-line lesion, a bilateral and usually widespread EEG abnormality

formation. Obviously a cortical 'lesion' will lead to a localised EEG disturbance, while one affecting cortical mid-line connections – for example, cortico-thalamic pathways – may cause a much widespread change which will nevertheless be lateralised. A 'lesion' affecting the mid-line structures causes bilateral disturbance which may also be widespread. These general principles apply whether the 'lesion' is of structural type, for example an intracerebral tumour, or dysfunctional, for example petit mal epilepsy. There are also combinations of structural and dysfunctional processes.

From the practical point of view we find that there are two main types of EEG abnormality: first, the 'structural', the continuous local usually delta disturbance characteristic of an intra-cerebral lesion; secondly, the 'dysfunctional', the episodic abnormality seen in epilepsy. In the former the background rhythms are disturbed continuously in the affected area, while in the latter, when the episodes subside, background activity can be seen to be unimpaired.

Sometimes abnormalities of either type are completely obvious, but on other occasions they are less convincing and here the technician is of great assistance. She is taught to spot the various features and then, by adjusting the controls of the machine and by connecting the electrodes in non-standard ways, to display the abnormality more clearly and convincingly. If there is muscle masking the potentials, this can be filtered out for part of the tracing. If there is a considerable quantity of low-frequency activity, on the other hand, the use of the low-frequency filters will in fact reduce the amount of slow activities but will allow assessment of faster elements in more detail. Another technique used to accentuate the slow activity is the use of a reduced paper speed. This, because it compresses the slow-wave activity, often makes it appear more prominent.

In subsequent chapters we shall be reconsidering the two basic types of abnormality, the 'structural' and the 'dysfunctional', in more detail, delineating the features which occur in various pathological processes and indicating, as far as possible, their specificity.

CHAPTER THREE

Cerebral Lesions (i) Cerebral Tumours

The EEG is of importance in the diagnosis of cerebral tumour (Walter 1936, Magnus *et al.* 1961, Decker and Knott 1972). Further, this subject illustrates many general principles of EEG, both practical and technical. First of all, the investigation is, from the patients' point of view, simple and painless, and it can easily be repeated on several occasions. Thus in patients suspected of cerebral tumour, for example because of the appearance of epilepsy in middle age, recordings can be carried out at three-monthly intervals, whereas it is quite inconceivable that neuro-radiological procedures would be repeated as frequently. In any case, these carry a definite risk in terms of morbidity and are more unpleasant for the patient. The EEG, with provisos, is a useful outpatient screening procedure if cerebral tumour is suspected. The chances of such an investigation being positive will be discussed later. However, and this is an important general principle in many conditions, a *negative* finding does not exclude the presence of a cerebral tumour. Another point is the non-specificity of EEG changes, which means that it is not often possible with certainty to distinguish between the EEG of a patient who has had a 'stroke' and one with a 'tumour'. Here the history, of course, is a differentiating factor, and the mnemonic CODE (condition, onset, duration and evolution) acts as a useful aid in neurological history taking.

The EEG findings

The key to the positive diagnosis of a cerebral tumour is a *continuous* local delta abnormality (Fischer-Williams *et al.* 1962). This type of activity is usually of high voltage and tends to be at the lower end of the delta range, that is at ½ to

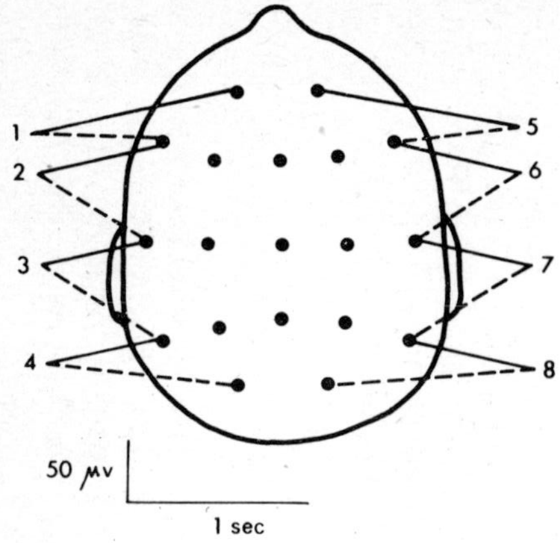

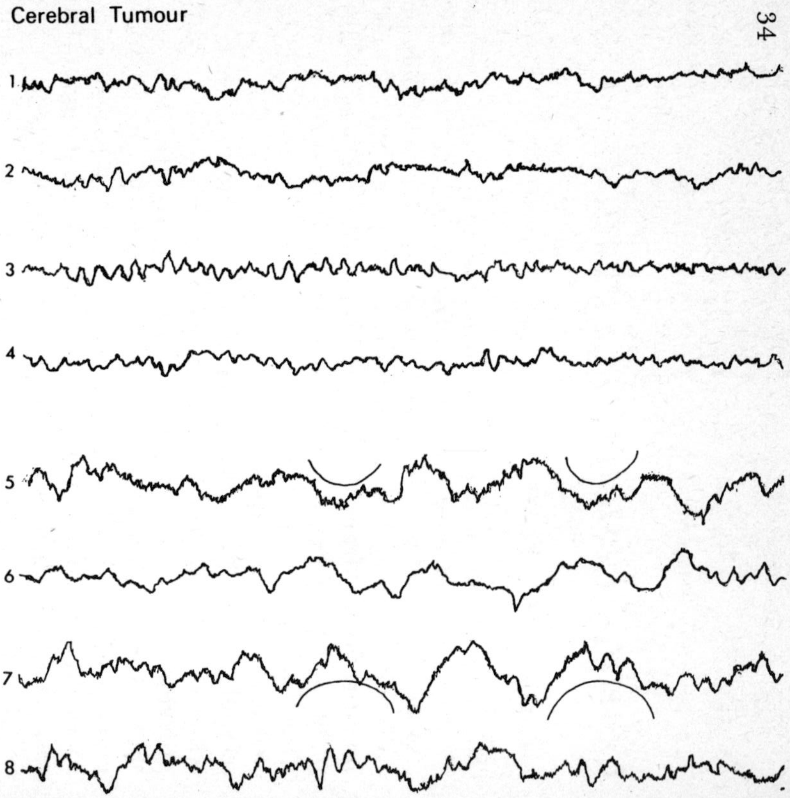

Figure 3.1 Shows an example of the changes which occur with cerebral tumour. There is extensive delta activity on the right side, while there is some preservation of background activity on the left. Note phase reversals between channels 5 and 7 (see text for detailed explanation, and Fig. 3.2 and 3.3); also the relatively lower amplitude of the disturbance in channel 6. Compare with the common average reference technique of recording on the same patient (Fig. 3.5)

Table 3.1 EEG changes seen in cerebral tumour patients

1. *Continuous* irregular *localised delta activity* usually of high voltage
2. Reduction of normal background rhythms such as alpha or beta activity
3. Sharp waves and spikes
4. Episodic bilateral rhythmic delta often frontal, in the presence of deep lesions and/or raised intracranial pressure. (The 'projected abnormality' or 'rhythm at a distance')

2 cycles per second (Table 3.1). Superimposed are components in the other frequency ranges appropriate for the area involved. The amounts of these vary from ample to absent (Fig. 3.1). In this latter case the possibility of an intracerebral abscess is raised (see Chapter 7). If the patient has a temporal lobe tumour, the amount of alpha activity on the side of the lesion is markedly reduced, of low amplitude and often slower than on the normal side, or it may be almost completely abolished. Another feature seen in the locality of the lesion is activity which may be loosely categorised as 'epileptic', i.e. spikes and sharp waves. These are interspersed with the delta activity and may occur in patients who have had epileptic seizures, as well as in those who have not. Generally, this type of activity is a feature of extracerebral and slowly growing intracerebral tumours, for example the meningioma and the oligodendroglioma.

The other main EEG feature seen in patients with cerebral tumour is Mono-rhythmic Sinusoidal Delta Activity (MSDA) or Frontal Intermittent Rhythmic Delta Activity (FIRDA), or, as I prefer to call it, simply bifrontal delta. This abnormality appears over both frontal lobes simultaneously and symmetrically, when there is a deeply placed lesion. It may often occur with raised intracranial pressure and in the absence of localised delta may indicate that the tumour is in the posterior fossa. Here the name 'rhythm at a distance' has been given, or sometimes a 'projected abnormality'. This type of episodic delta is an example of the dysfunctional abnormality referred to in Chapter 2, since as in the example given here there is not necessarily a lesion in the frontal lobes. When bifrontal delta is seen, the EEG must be interpreted with care, for it can also occur in patients following a series of epileptic fits, in drowsy patients with a metabolic or toxic confusional state and in many other conditions. In our experience (Rowan *et al.* 1974) it is of greatest significance in relation to a space-occupying process when seen in alert patients. Then, it strongly suggests that there is an intracerebral lesion, whereas it may be seen in drowsy patients who have a marked metabolic and electrolyte disturbance due to multiple systemic metastases but without any definite lesion in the brain.

Factors affecting EEG abnormality

There are a number of factors which affect the presence and the amount of EEG abnormality (Table 3.2). The most important is probably the size of the lesion (Strang and Marsan 1961). With tumours less than 2.5 centimetres in diameter the tracing may be quite normal. If the tumour has caused seizures, its size may be smaller than this and still show EEG features. The site of the lesion is also of

Table 3.2 Factors affecting the EEG findings in cerebral tumour patients

1. Size	No abnormality usually seen with lesions less than 2.5 centimetres in diameter (unless seizures have occurred)
2. Site	Supratentorial lesions more readily produce EEG abnormality than those in the infratentorial situation
3. Depth	Deep seated lesions cause widespread non-localised, 'projected' abnormality. Superficial lesions cause localised disturbance with phase reversal or flattening (see text)
4. Pathology	Malignant intracerebral tumours are more likely to produce EEG abnormality than benign extracerebral tumours. Slow growing intracerebral lesions cause spikes and sharp waves
5. Rate of growth	The faster the progress of the tumour the more likely is EEG abnormality to be seen, especially if there is sudden bleed or cyst formation
6. Raised intracranial pressure	Leads to generalised episodic EEG abnormality in the absence of focal features, but slowing of background rhythms
7. Disturbance in level of consciousness	Gives rise to widespread bilateral changes possibly with false localising features

significance. In general, lesions in the posterior fossa are less readily detected by EEG investigation. These lesions may cause disturbance in the recording remote from their actual site, for example over the frontal or occipital areas. The depth of the lesion is also of importance. The more deeply placed it is, the more widespread is the abnormality because of the interruption of cortico-mid-line connections. Deeply placed lesions also tend to produce projected abnormalities, for example bifrontal delta which may obscure some less clearly defined localising features. Superficial lesions, on the other hand, tend to cause localised suppression of activity and in addition phase reversal (see below). A sleep recording may be helpful in defining the 'depth' of the tumour (Silverman and Groff 1957).

The histological nature of the tumour is of prime importance. Malignant intracerebral tumours, especially those which are rapidly expanding, produce marked abnormality. On the whole, extracerebral lesions such as meningiomas do not produce early EEG change, although this may be seen if epilepsy supervenes. The nature of the abnormality caused by meningiomas is somewhat different from that observed with intracerebral tumours. The type of pattern is often described as 'irritative' since there may be augmentation of the normal types of activity appropriate for the particular areas. Thus, there may be an increase in the amount of beta and mu activity if an irritative lesion is situated in the fronto-rolandic areas, while the alpha may be augmented in amplitude with a more posterior siting of such a lesion.

As with many other types of lesion, the more rapid the progress the greater the chance that the EEG will be abnormal. Thus an expanding tumour causes abnormality, while an atrophic process may show remarkably little EEG change. If there is raised intracranial pressure consciousness tends to be disturbed, but this is usually a late feature in patients with cerebral tumours, and when it occurs it leads to widespread bilateral changes in the EEG which may mask the localised abnormality. These may be revealed after surgical decompression, or ventricular drainage, and sometimes after steroids or mannitol, which reduce intracranial pressure. So a repeat tracing can be helpful.

Early signs of a intracranial tumour

The EEG, like skull X-rays and the isotope brain scan, is an investigation that can be carried out readily without admission to hospital. It is therefore of importance to have some idea of the likelihood of positive diagnosis of cerebral tumour so that decisions can be made about admission for

Table 3.3 Early EEG signs in cerebral tumour patient, for example on initial outpatient referral

Glioma	Usually positive
Meningioma	May be negative if no epileptic seizures
Metastases	Positive if lesion more than 2.5 centimetres in diameter
Posterior fossa tumours	Only 30% positive
Special tumours	Acoustic neuromas, tumours around foramen magnum, in pituitary fossa – EEG negative or non-specific features only

further investigations (Table 3.3). With a malignant glioma the EEG is usually positive, while with a meningioma it may often be negative. The isotope brain scan is obviously an important supplementary investigation here because it usually shows a striking area of uptake in a meningioma case. When metastatic deposits are suspected the EEG may be positive, but it should be borne in mind that until the lesion or lesions reach the size of 2.5 centimetres diameter, unless they happen to be strategically placed, no very specific EEG abnormality will appear. When the tumour is located in the posterior fossa a proportion of EEGs may be negative or show essentially non-specific features. Similarly, with tumours such as acoustic neuromas or those in the pituitary fossa, the EEG may be quite normal or only show very minor changes. One special condition in which the EEG may be helpful is in patients with recurrent tumours; for example, a meningioma may have been removed with success and later the patient begins again to complain of headache or other non-specific symptoms. Ordinarily, the tracing will revert to normal in a patient following surgery for a meningioma, and abnormal findings a year or so later strongly suggest recurrence. However, if the EEG is going to be used in this way it is advisable to carry out a post-operative EEG about three months after discharge from hospital, so that this will form a base line for comparison when there is a later suggestion of recurrence on clinical grounds (Prior 1968).

Localisation in the EEG

Localisation of a lesion on the basis of the EEG is best thought of in two separate stages; first, the 'electrical localisation', and secondly, the relationship this bears to the actual anatomical localisation.

To understand the electrical phenomena we must re-capitulate the way in which the EEG electrodes are connected to the apparatus to produce the multi-channel recording. Each amplifying system for a channel has two inputs, the active and the indifferent, and the write-out is the difference in potential between these two. In the EEG Convention the active input is always termed the 'black lead' and the indifferent, the 'white lead'. The amplifying system is arranged such that a negative voltage affecting the 'black lead' causes an upward deflection in the channel. A mnemonic for this is Black Upward Negative – BUN. Conversely a negative potential affecting the white lead will cause a downward deflection; positive voltages obviously having the reverse effects.

Now consider a specific bipolar array. It is usual to link adjacent electrodes from either front to back or side to side across the head. The general plan of such a bipolar arrangement involving three electrodes is shown in Fig. 3.2. The first electrode in the chain forms a black lead for Channel A and the second electrode, the white lead for that channel. In addition the second electrode is connected to the next channel, Channel B, as the black lead and the third electrode to the white lead of that channel. Therefore any discharge arising in the neighbourhood of the second electrode will have the opposite effects in channels A and B, the deflections pointing towards one another indicating the site of the discharge. This phenomemon is called a 'phase reversal' and is the key to electrical localisation on bipolar recording.

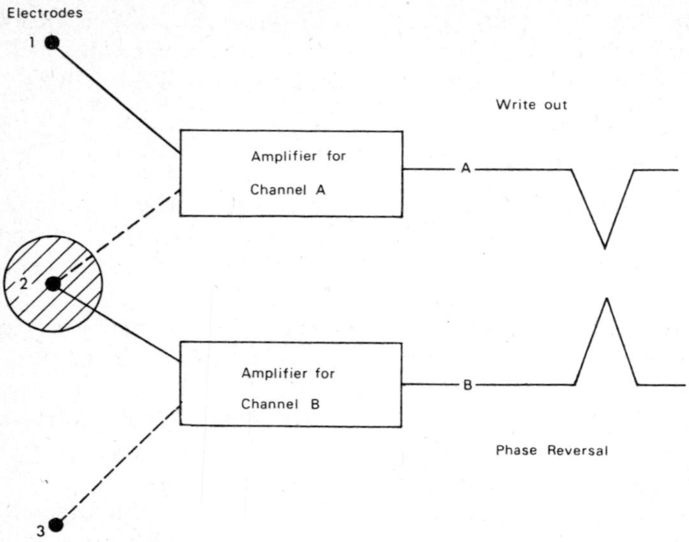

Figure 3.2 Shows how a phase reversal arises. The hatched area around electrode 2 represents area of negative potential arising from a lesion, e.g. a tumour. This electrode is connected to the white grid (dotted lines) of channel A and the black grid (solid lines) of channel B. See text for further explanation

If a phase reversal is present then the disturbance is described as 'focal'.

Of course we cannot locate a point merely by bearings taken in one plane, so as in cartography, so in electroencephalography phase reversals are looked for ideally in two directions at right angles. It is the principle of quadrangulation, the technique used in pin-pointing a location on a map.

There is another point also. If we have a discharge which affects two adjacent electrodes equally on bipolar recording, the channel connected to these two electrodes will show no deflection whatsoever, that is, it will appear 'flat' (Fig. 3.3).

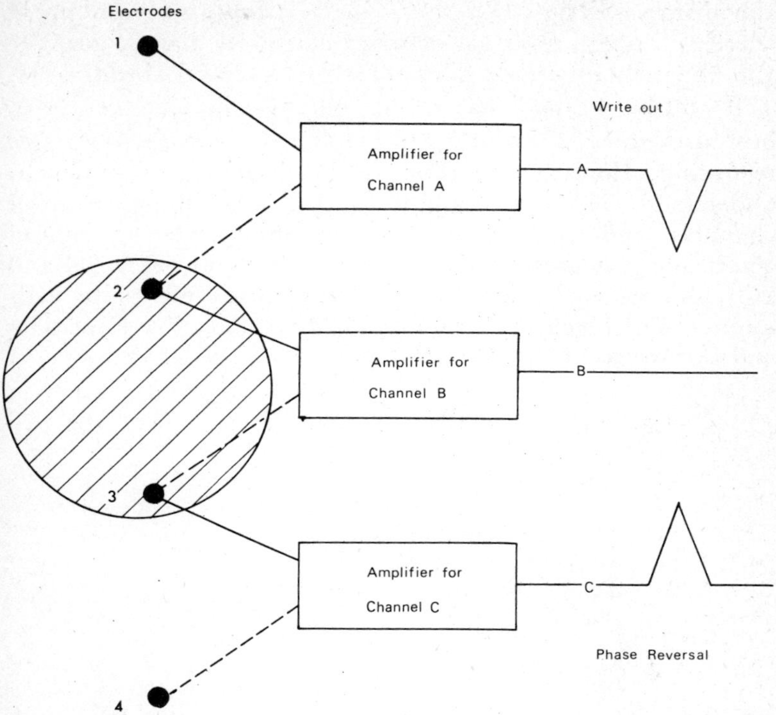

Figure 3.3 An elaboration of the features seen in Fig. 3.2. Here a much larger area of potential arising from a lesion affects mainly two adjacent electrodes (2 and 3) equally. Thus the output from channel B is a straight line. In actual practice it is more often an area of relative 'flattening' as is seen in Fig. 3.1 channel 6

This is very confusing for the beginner but can perhaps be clarified by a simple analogy. In a schoolboy game two boys stand back to back, their elbows linked, the aim of each being to get the other's feet off the ground. Imagine a pointer attached to the head of one of them and any movement seen regarded as an EEG write-out. If there is no movement of the pointer this could be due either to their merely standing with their elbows linked or to their applying equal and opposite forces to each other. We can prove that even in the state of 'no movement' there is a force being applied, for if one boy suddenly unlinks his elbows the other is sent flying off into the distance. Thus, a flat channel on bipolar recording, if there is a phase reversal occurring across it, that is, between the channels on either side, constitutes a focal abnormality.

It will be recalled that we use, not just bipolar recording, but also some form of mono-polar or average reference recording. Here the method of localisation is simpler to understand. The deflection is in the same direction in all channels and the channel which shows the maximum amplitude is nearest to the source of discharge (Figs. 3.4 and 3.5). Of course, the same convention of black and white leads applies. The black leads are attached to the active electrodes and the white to the reference point such as the earlobe; or,

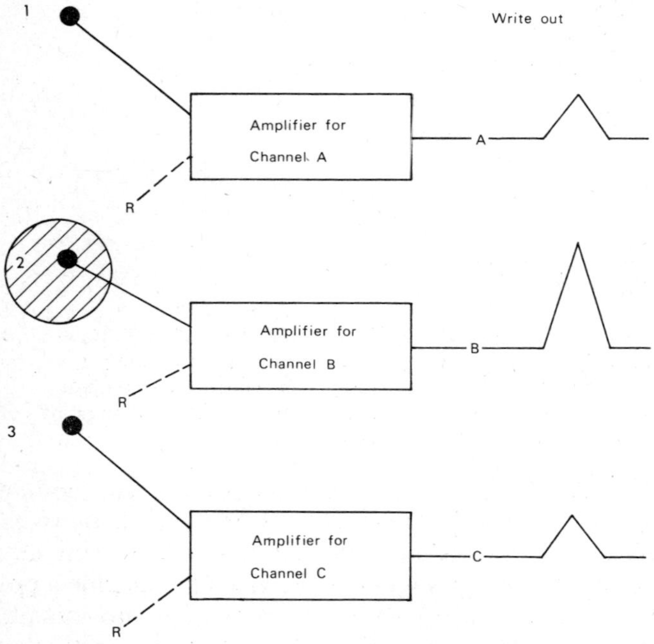

Figure 3.4 Shows the effect of using a reference electrode which is connected to the white grid of each channel. Here the height of the deflection indicates the electrode which is nearest the source of potential, the hatched area. A clinical example of this is demonstrated in Fig. 3.5

in the other reference technique – common average reference – the white lead is formed by the sum of potentials from all the scalp electrodes. The bipolar and monopolar recording techniques are best used together to get maximum information on 'electrical' localisation, and the techniques apply also to other phenomena, including (see Chapter 4) sharp waves and spikes, as well as to the slow-wave discharges discussed here.

Turning now to anatomical localisation, it is important to emphasise the patho-physiological basis of the characteristic continuous high-voltage delta activity. This is produced by oedema of the relatively normal neurones at the periphery of the tumour. The tumour itself is electrically silent, and when it approaches the cortex a local area of diminished activity is found. Sometimes, if the cortex is destroyed, an area of 'electrical silence' is seen. This area of silence of course should be contrasted with the 'flat channel' described when recording is by bipolar techniques. When there is a genuine area of flattening, confirmed by monopolar recording, the electrical and the clinical localisation correspond and the tumour is very superficial. If high-voltage delta activity displays phase reversals, the tumour is relatively superficial. More deep seated tumours show relatively wide areas of delta without phase reversal. Then the maximum EEG abnormality may be at some distance from the centre of the tumour, leading to a discrepancy between the EEG and clinical localisation. There is also a tendency for tumours to be located in the EEG more laterally and more posteriorly than they are in the anatomical sense. Nevertheless, bearing all these difficulties in mind, EEG localisation of tumours may be almost as exact as those with neuro-radiological investigations (Van der Drift 1957), though for precise anatomical localisation neuro-radiological investigations are usually necessary. The main use of the EEG, however, is as a preliminary screening procedure which can be done without any risk.

Cerebral tumour and other space-occupying lesions

Of course, the principles of localisation mentioned here apply

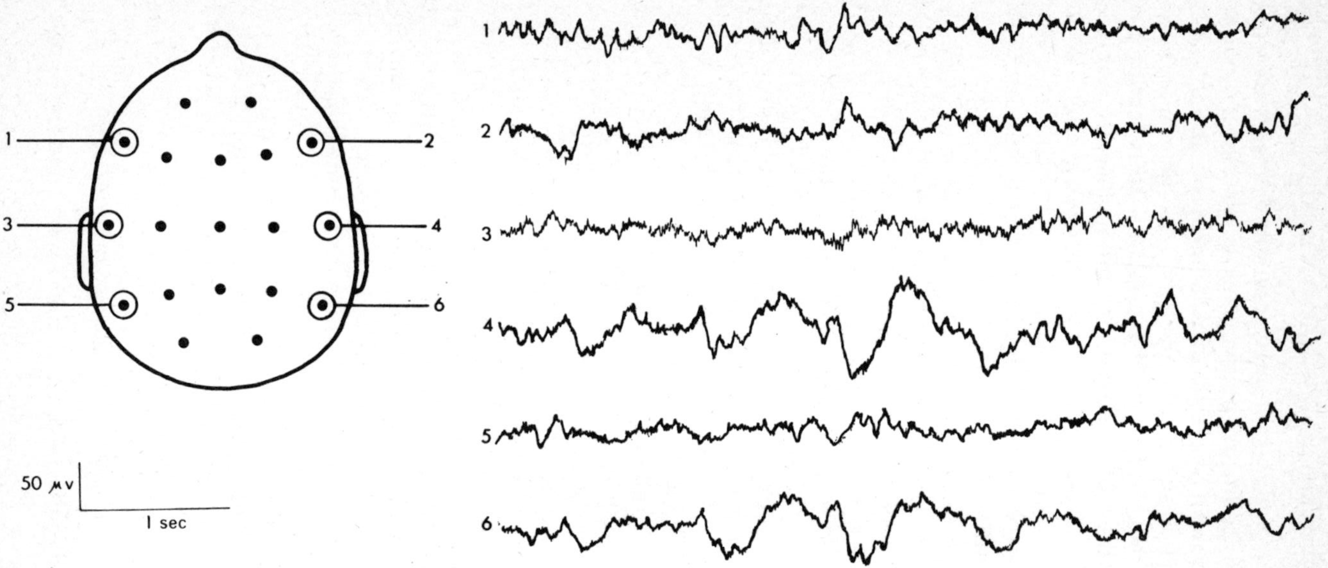

Figure 3.5 Common average reference recording. The channels are arranged alternately, those with even numbers from the right side. Notice the maximum deflection is in channel 4 indicating that the mid-temporal electrode is nearest to the source of the electrical disturbance. Note that this corresponds to the localisation by phase reversal shown in Fig. 3.1. Each system points to the same electrode as being nearest to the source of the discharge confirming that this is its definite electrical origin

to other types of lesion, and in subsequent chapters we shall consider lesions due to cerebro-vascular disease, e.g. haematomas, and infections, such as cerebral abscess and ones due to head injury. There are some differences in EEG terms in the morphology of the phenomena seen which can help to distinguish between them even when the recording is studied 'blind', that is without reference to the clinical material. Though exact differentiation of these EEG features is for the specialist, some of them will be discussed in later chapters (see Fig. 5.2).

In conclusion, it can be seen that the EEG is of value for the assessment of 'tumour suspects'. Positive findings are of great importance, as is shown in a recent study of 149 patients reported by Decker and Knott (1972): 19 of the patients had positive EEG findings on their initial examination, and this preceded the clinico-pathological diagnosis by at least a year; in other words in that study positive EEG findings were not taken seriously. If there is doubt in the mind of the clinician, follow-up EEGs at three- or six-monthly intervals can be helpful, the EEG usually showing an increasing abnormality as the pathological *process* advances.

CHAPTER FOUR

Epilepsy

Epilepsy is an important and interesting condition for the electroencephalographer and one in which he contributes significantly to establishing the diagnosis. In many departments, one third of all referrals will be in some way related to this condition. There are many reasons for these referrals (see Table 4.1). The clinician seeks help in the diagnosis of petit mal and other forms of epileptic attack, in the surveillance of patients with late onset epilepsy, or in considering the suitability for the surgical treatment of epilepsy. Doubt has been cast on the use of the EEG in epilepsy (Matthews 1973, Pappworth 1974), and so in the course of this chapter I shall give some indication of what can and what cannot be expected from the test. The critical point, which needs constant emphasis, is the fact that epilepsy is a *clinical diagnosis;* and a detailed history with an eye-witness account of what actually happened and what followed the attack, for example post-ictal confusion, will usually give greater information than a single routine tracing long after the event.

Table 4.1 Use of the EEG in patients with epilepsy

1. Confirmation of diagnosis
2. Type of epilepsy, e.g. petit mal
3. Presence or absence of underlying lesion, e.g. brain tumour
4. Location of the focus or foci
5. Presence of trigger factors, e.g. light sensitivity in television epilepsy
6. Presence or absence of associated brain disease
7. Effectiveness of anticonvulsant medication (including monitoring during status epilepticus), indication of anticonvulsant intoxication
8. Suitability of patient for surgical treatment

Epilepsy is a complex disorder because there are difficulties of definition and classification, manifold psycho-social problems (see, for example, Scott 1973), and in addition uncertainties about the basic cause. From the clinical point of view, epilepsy can be defined simply as a tendency to recurring seizures. A somewhat wider definition, however, is required, and the following suffices: 'Epilepsy is a sudden and usually repeated behavioural change associated with impairment of consciousness lasting seconds or minutes, accompanied by abnormal electrical discharge in the brain.' These discharges can almost always be seen in the scalp EEG, their character reflecting the basic patho-physiology. This is beginning to be better understood, mainly as a result of studies in animals using intracerebral recordings of experimentally induced epilepsy. The epileptic phenomena arise because of instability of cell membranes of particular neurones, leading to sudden rapid and excessive neuronal discharges which are prolonged and spread rapidly. In the scalp recording, spikes are the basic phenomena, and these appear in a generalised fashion during convulsions. The spike relates to the excitatory phase. Once again, considering the scalp recording, slow wave activity or flattening is seen following a convulsion, and this relates to the inhibitory phase. In petit mal we see a combination of the spike and the slow wave, the two being paired in a regular fashion. This can be viewed simply as a condition in which inhibition builds up appropriately, preventing a minor attack becoming a major one.

Classification of epilepsy

Turning to the question of classification, this ideally has to take into account, not only the basic cause, but also the seizure type. A simple classification into 'idiopathic' and 'symptomatic' epilepsy has something to recommend it. The diagnosis of idiopathic epilepsy implies a seizure without an aura, lack of evidence of a CNS lesion, particular EEG features, and possibly a family history of fits. The label symptomatic, on the other hand, means seizures, possibly with an aura, and focal components, particular EEG features which are different from those in idiopathic epilepsy, and possibly a history of a CNS insult, and perhaps abnormal neurological signs. There is generally no family history of fits. Another form of symptomatic epilepsy, usually non-focal, occurs in patients who have metabolic, toxic or other disorders which lead to secondary brain dysfunction; for example, a patient with renal failure developing generalised seizures during the course of the illness.

The seizures in idiopathic epilepsy are generalised and include grand mal and petit mal; symptomatic seizures are focal or partial, although they may become generalised, and an aura usually occurs. However, in some instances there is no aura and the seizures are generalised from the start. This shows that there is an overlap with idiopathic epilepsy – a feature which indicates the difficulties of classification.

From the EEG point of view, another simple sub-division into centrencephalic (or primary sub-cortical) and focal cortical epilepsy is useful. The former corresponds to generalised seizures and the label 'idiopathic', the latter to 'symptomatic' epilepsy. An amalgam of these classifications is shown in Table 4.2, but whichever is used there is always a group which have to be labelled 'unclassifiable'. None the less, some system is essential for everyday work, and in my view the simpler it is the better.

Table 4.2 A classification of epilepsy

Type	1. Idiopathic generalised	2. Symptomatic	3. Unclassified
Fit pattern	Petit mal Grand mal Myoclonic	Usually focal or partial, i.e. temporal lobe (psychomotor), Jacksonian; can be generalised	Inconstant
EEG	'Subcortical' 'centrencephalic'	Focal, cortical	Various

(Based on Merlis, J.K., 'Proposal for an International Classification of Epilepsy,' *Epilepsia* (1970) *11*, 114-19).

From the purely clinical point of view it is sometimes useful to have a sub-category which is labelled 'late onset epilepsy' with an arbitary starting point of age 20 or 25 years. This group contains a much larger proportion of the patients with symptomatic epilepsy and in whom there is an underlying structural abnormality, which in a certain percentage may be of an expanding nature. In these cases, as we shall see later, serial EEG recordings can be very useful. Another aspect of classification concerns communication with others working in the field and a considerable amount of effort has recently been devoted to establishing an acceptable international system, although as yet it has not been generally accepted.

Origin and spread of the epileptic discharge

We are still left with a problem of where the epileptic discharge arises and how it spreads in both centrencephalic and focal cortical epilepsy (Brazier 1973). There are no definite answers to these questions, but it is clear from experimental work that epileptic discharges can be produced by stimulation of the non-specific thalamic nuclei and the reticular formation. This suggests a mid-line origin for centrencephalic discharge which in the scalp EEG presents synchronously over homologous cortical areas (Fig. 4.1) and can be recorded spreading via thalamic cortical pathways; while a focal cortical discharge in the motor area may remain relatively localised and lead to clinical changes appropriate to its site, for example, twitching of the thumb. However, not only may such focal phenomena spread to involve other areas of the motor cortex (the Jacksonian type), but in some instances there is an even wider change leading to a generalised seizure, implying that both hemispheres have become involved. How has the discharge spread to the other hemisphere? Through the corpus callosum? In favour of this view is the evidence from corpus callosal section for the treatment of epilepsy. In some patients this leads to relief of generalised seizures. Penfield (1969) puts forward a different view. He suggests that cortical discharges 'fire' into the brain stem grey matter, and then secondarily 'bombard' both cerebral hemispheres. In fact the pattern in the scalp EEG of such cases of secondary generalised epilepsy is very similar to that in centrencephalic epilepsy, so that on this score at least, Penfield's view seems tenable.

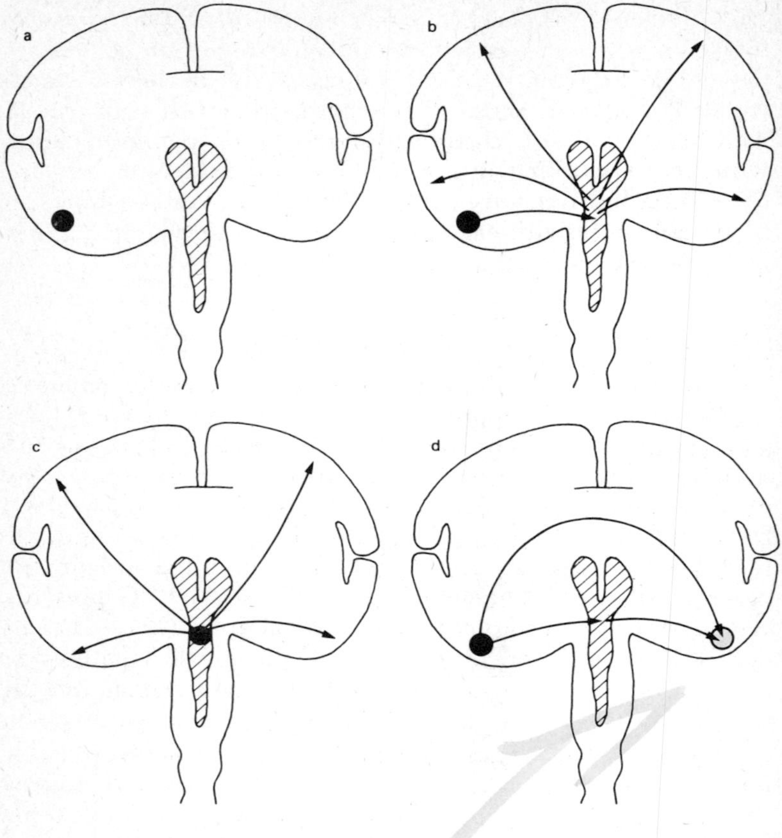

Figure 4.1 Hypothetical models of the origin and spread of epileptic discharges. The hatched portion represents the thalamus and reticular formation. The darkened circle represents an epileptic discharge

(a) A discharge which remains localised as in some forms of Jacksonian and temporal lobe epilepsy

(b) A localised discharge spreading to the mid-line structures and leading to subsequent generalised discharge; the so-called secondary subcortical epilsepy

(c) The situation in primary generalised epilepsy, whether it is of petit mal or grand mal type. Here it is hypothesised that the discharge begins in the mid-line structures and spreads in a generalised fashion

(d) Here a localised discharge impinges on homologous areas of the opposite hemisphere. The possible routes are either through the corpus callosum or through other mid-line structures. After many years a 'mirror' focus (see text) appears and then this takes over independently

The EEG during seizures

So much for the theory. Now let us turn to the EEG features in the patient. These can best be divided into 'ictal', i.e. those accompanying a fit, and the 'inter-ictal,' i.e. those seen between attacks. Considering the ictal changes, we should emphasise that the time spent by the patient in the EEG department is of the order of three quarters of an hour for a routine tracing, and, of that time, perhaps just over a half is actual recording. It is obvious, therefore, that even if a patient is having one attack a day, the chances of recording during a seizure are very small. This applies particularly to major fits, though it is somewhat more common to record during temporal lobe attacks, and much the most frequent disorder in which attacks are witnessed and recorded is from patients with petit mal. These patients often have many attacks in the course of a single day.

The EEG during a seizure shows repetitive spikes. In the convulsive or grand mal attack these spikes are generalised (see Fig. 4.2) at the start, whereas in a temporal lobe seizure the ictal discharge may remain quite localised, and in petit mal each spike is regularly followed by a slow wave.

The technician, because she sees a fit perhaps every week, learns to recognise the clinical features which occur while the recording is in progress. Of particular interest is the tracing annotated by the technician, so that we can follow not only the development of the electrical phenomena but the timing of the various parts of the attack, as well as the total duration. Of course this can be done with a stop-watch, but the clinician or nurse may not have one handy, and in any case, because the EEG technician sees many seizures, she becomes adept at describing them. Thus the patient may appear to be frightened for a moment or two before any movement or jerkings occur. From the tracing, which runs usually at the speed of 3 centimeters per second, we can estimate that the 'aura' or warning, which coincides with the very beginning of the electrical discharge, lasts a second or so and that the overall duration of the fit is two minutes. It is also possible to estimate the duration of post-ictal confusion.

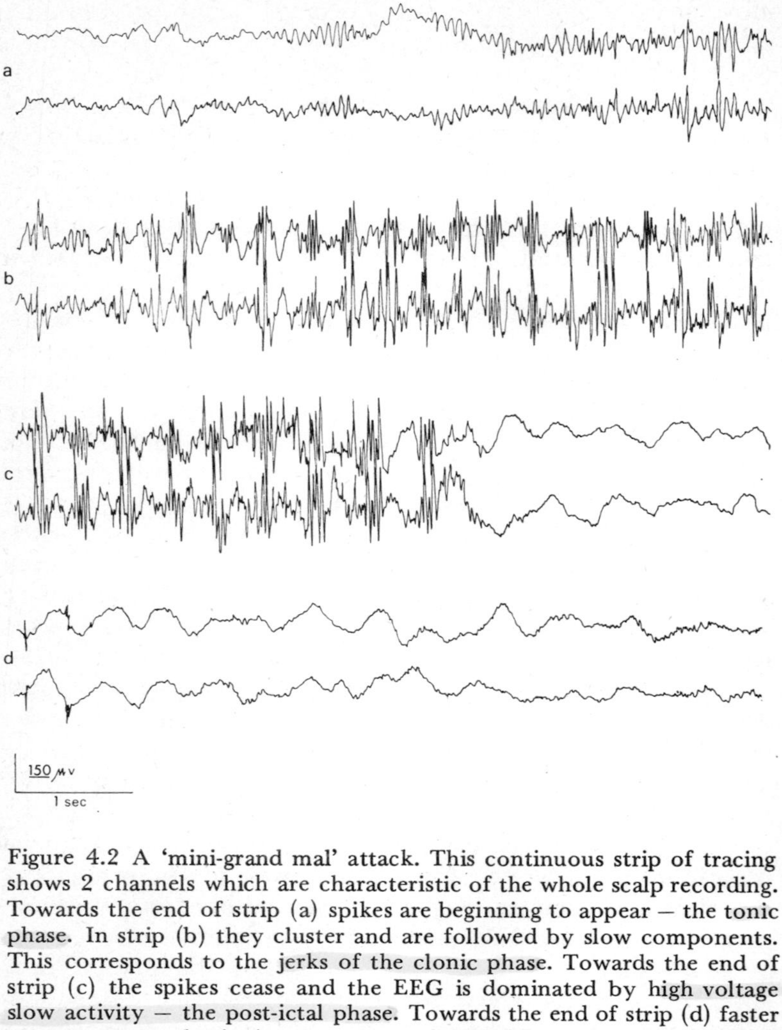

Figure 4.2 A 'mini-grand mal' attack. This continuous strip of tracing shows 2 channels which are characteristic of the whole scalp recording. Towards the end of strip (a) spikes are beginning to appear – the tonic phase. In strip (b) they cluster and are followed by slow components. This corresponds to the jerks of the clonic phase. Towards the end of strip (c) the spikes cease and the EEG is dominated by high voltage slow activity – the post-ictal phase. Towards the end of strip (d) faster components are beginning to return and the EEG corresponds almost to the early part of strip (a). Note the high voltage of the discharges. This EEG was recorded with amplification of 150 microvolts per centimetre. (Most illustrations in this book are at a third of this amplification)

Let us first consider the grand mal or convulsive attack and its electrographic concomitants. Because of the muscle and movement during the seizure, it is rarely possible to obtain a satisfactory scalp recording. However, many attacks have been monitored using implanted or subdural electrodes. The technique requires the neurosurgeon to make burr holes and insert a leash of sterilised wires into or over various areas suspected, on clinical grounds, of being the source of the attacks. This method is usually employed when there is doubt about the diagnosis of epilepsy or when a patient is under consideration for surgery because of intractable seizures.

Just before the grand mal attack, low-voltage fast activity appears and increases in amplitude, a change which lasts a few seconds and then gives way to generalised high-amplitude spikes. These occur in the tonic phase of the seizure, and as it proceeds there is a tendency for the spikes to increase in amplitude but to diminish in frequency. The clonic phase is heralded by the appearance of grouped spikes corresponding to the clonic spasms, separated by slow waves. As these spasms diminish, so the spikes become less and less frequent, until finally they disappear, leaving the characteristic low-amplitude post-ictal record. What scanty activity does appear is at the lower end of the delta range. The delta activity then increases in frequency, and over the next few minutes or hours a more normal EEG pattern emerges. Episodic bifrontal delta activity and general disorganisation of the tracing may, however, persist for as long as 24 to 48 hours.

The temporal lobe attack is somewhat different (see Table 4.3). The first change noted in the EEG, and this precedes any behavioural alteration, may be the disappearance of the inter-ictal spike and sharp wave discharges. Even before any definite ictal phenomena can be seen in the scalp EEG, the alpha may attenuate, presumably as the patient becomes aware of 'internal change' – the warning or aura of the attack. Quite rapidly a number of 'electrical' phenomena appear; sometimes definite spikes are seen in a localised fashion. At other times rhythmic smooth outlined activity is obvious or sometimes spike and wave discharges. These have a much more rapid repetition rate and a lower amplitude than those appearing in patients with petit mal (see below).

Table 4.3 Temporal lobe attack

	Behaviour	EEG
Before attack	Normal	Isolated L. temporal sharp waves
Attack begins	Opens eyes, looks worried. Flushed, dilated pupils	Sharp waves disappear Low-voltage fast activity L. temporal region
10 secs later	Head turns to left	High-voltage repetitive sharp waves in L. temporal region
10 secs later	Unresponsive to commands	Widespread sharp waves and delta over both hemispheres
20 secs later	Resists attempts to keep head on pillow	Continuous spikes in L. temporal region
20 secs later	Lies quietly	Spikes continue L. temporal region Sharp waves and delta elsewhere
40 secs later	Attempts to get up from couch, smiles, but is confused	Mainly muscle artefact
50 secs later	Patient still confused but co-operative	Reverted to pre-attack pattern with alpha activity on both sides and L. temporal sharp waves.

As the fit proceeds, the discharge, of whatever type, increases in amplitude, while decreasing in frequency. Thus rhythmic activity of 4 to 8 cycles per second may be widely seen over both hemispheres as the attack develops. The discharge is usually asymmetrical, being of higher amplitude over the hemisphere in which the seizure began. Sometimes the discharge disappears quite suddenly, leaving a relatively featureless record, but at other times it diminishes, becoming intermingled with the delta components. As the background elements return a definite asymmetry is usually noted, and the activity is reduced over the hemisphere in which the attack commenced. On rare occasions, though behavioural phenomena are seen during a seizure, little change occurs in the recording itself. None the less, in these circumstances when the attack ceases a definite asymmetry of alpha and/or fast components may be obvious, confirming at least the hemisphere in which the attack started.

'Non-epilepsy'

The fact that there are almost always manifestations in the EEG during a seizure helps in the positive diagnosis of 'non-epilepsy'. Fairly frequently, perhaps once a month, we are asked to record the EEG of a patient who is having frequent attacks in the ward and the appearances of which suggest that they are not occurring on an epileptic basis. In these circumstances, though the tracing itself during the attack may be marred by muscle and movement artefact, the re-appearance immediately after the attack of normal rhythms bilaterally and symmetrically strongly suggests that the 'attacks' are not seizures.

This, of course, is a complex subject because, in addition to patients who have attacks which are definitely and constantly hysterical, there are a small number of epileptic patients who seem to have both epileptic and non-epileptic attacks. Apart from the EEG support of a clinical hunch about the nature of the attacks, it is important in these patients to look for positive evidence of psycho-social disturbance which could account for the appearance of functional episodes. Absence of organic features alone is not sufficient for the diagnosis of 'non-epilepsy'.

EEG changes between fits

There are EEG changes which, though they occur between fits, strongly support a clinical diagnosis of epilepsy (see Table 4.4). These inter-ictal changes in the EEGs of patients with generalised seizures include brief widespread bursts of

Table 4.4 Inter-ictal features

Hard 'signs'	Bursts of spike and wave activity (see Table 4.5 for different types)
	Bursts of generalised spikes
	Focal spikes or sharp waves
	Localised sharp/slow complexes
Soft 'signs'	Disorganised background with excess of diffuse slow activity
	Episodic generalised or localised slow activity
	Rhythmic posterior delta activity
	Localised sharpened theta activity

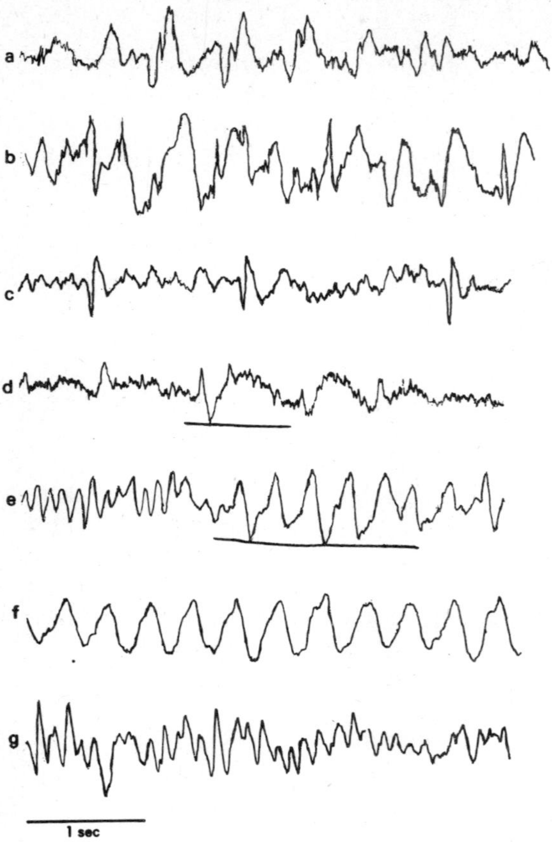

spike and wave. They do not have a smooth regular outline of the 3 cycle per second spike and wave seen in petit mal; they also tend to have many spike elements and a faster or slower repetition rate (See Table 4.4 and Fig. 4.3). The tracings of patients with myoclonic epilepsy show bursts of generalised spikes followed by slow waves. All the changes may first appear with, or may be enhanced by, overbreathing (Morgan and Scott 1970). Patients who have seizures in front of a television set show discharges of spikes and waves during photic stimulation. Recently Binnie *et al.* (1973) have used an actual television set in the recording suite and have found

Figure 4.3 Inter-ictal EEG changes. They may be localised or generalised and are of varying amplitude
(a) A run of irregular spike and wave activity which was seen over both frontal regions
(b) A slightly more prolonged run of irregular spike and wave visible over one occipital region
(c) Individual sharp waves occurring in the left rolandic region
(d) A sharp/slow complex (underlined) followed by two slightly dissimilar complexes. These occurred over the left temporal region in a patient having temporal lobe attacks
(e) An episode of delta activity (underlined) which was seen in a high voltage and generalised fashion. Note the normal alpha activity occurring before this episode
(f) A run of rhythmic delta activity seen over both posterior head regions in a more or less symmetrical fashion, from a patient with petit mal epilepsy
(g) Part of a disorganised EEG. Alpha, theta and delta activities are intermingled. This was observed over both posterior head regions in a patient with chronic 'epilepsy'

that it is effective for eliciting EEG abnormality in patients with idiopathic epilepsy who have not had television-induced seizures.

The characteristic features of inter-ictal EEG of patients with focal cortical epilepsy are spikes or sharp waves or localised complexes of sharp and slow waves. These are usually frequent and localised, for example to the anterior or mid temporal region in patients who have temporal lobe epilepsy. Quite often I am asked what is the difference between a spike and a sharp wave. In practical terms the answer is 'nothing' because they are both the same basic neurophysiological phenomenon. Descriptively, however, a spike is a disturbance of briefer duration (less than 80 milliseconds) and therefore has a sharper outline that the sharp wave which lasts from 80 to 200 milliseconds.

There are other inter-ictal changes which are less specific, listed as 'soft signs' in Table 4.4 and 4.5. These consist, for example, of disorganisation of background activity and generalised episodes of theta and delta activity. Once again, these changes are exaggerated during overbreathing. However, it should be emphasised that such features may appear in a variety of other conditions, so that they must be interpreted with care in patients who have a dubious history of epilepsy.

Table 4.5 Types of spike and wave, classified by repetition rate

Type	Repetition rate	Seizures	Occurrence in referral population	Mentation
Typical	3/sec	Petit mal occasional grand mal	Uncommon	Normal
Atypical	2/sec (slow)	Grand mal and various minor attacks	Frequent	Subnormal
	4/sec	Grand mal	Very frequent	Normal or 'slow'.
	6/sec (fast)	May not have seizures	Rare	Psychosis or normal

So far I have rarely used the word 'paroxysmal'. This by international definition refers to almost any type of phenomenon which stands out from the on-going activity. It can be a spike or sharp wave complex or a run of slow components. Thus 'paroxysmal' could be applied to both the definite and the indefinite inter-ictal changes. Because this is an important distinction I tend to avoid the term 'paroxysmal' in the conclusion of EEG reports. Nevertheless it is commonly used, and then it is important to determine what exactly was seen in the EEG. If it was a definite discharge containing spikes, it strongly supports a clinical diagnosis of epilepsy; if merely episodic slow, the EEG must be interpreted with care in the light of the history and the physical signs.

Of course, the EEG of a patient with a structural abnormality, such as an expanding glioma, shows continuous localised slow activity having the characteristics described in Chapter 3. Sometimes, however, the patient with an atrophic lesion may show few changes after a series of fits. Hence a repeat record some days later is often of value in such cases.

Petit mal

Petit mal, although well recognised, is a relatively uncommon kind of epilepsy. It occurs in childhood; other types of epilepsy in this age group will be dealt with in Chapter 8. The importance of petit mal to the electroencephalographer is the generalised spike and wave complexes which appear with a regular repetition rate of 3 per second (see Fig. 4.4) and these are as nearly diagnostic of epilepsy as any EEG feature can be. The recording of the typical patient shows many bursts of spike and wave with varying length. Some, the longer, are accompanied by fluttering of eyelids or minor limb-jerkings, others by more profound disturbances in tone. It may increase or decrease, although they may not necessarily be detected during the EEG as the patient is lying on the couch (Penry 1973). Some of the briefer bursts do not seem to be accompanied by any behavioural change at all in the patient. They would then be regarded as 'inter-ictal'. If particular care is taken to look for minor alterations in the level of mental functioning during the recording, some appear to be accompanied by a change. For example, if the patient is asked to count or tap regularly with a finger on a book, she may hesitate when a brief burst of spike and wave occurs, even if only of a second's duration. However, with such simple tasks no disturbance in mentation may be found. Then it is necessary to increase the task difficulty to demonstrate it. The patient may have to be asked to count backwards in twos from a hundred, and a burst of spike and wave may suddenly cause interruption in the counting. Sometimes many such increments in the testing are necessary before any change is seen (Hutt *et al.* 1972). On occasions none can be demonstrated. Thus the spike and wave discharges may be either ictal or inter-ictal.

Three cycle per second spike and wave is sometimes called 'primary bilateral synchrony', because the disturbance appears symmetrically, with the same timing over the two hemispheres and without focal discharges at any stage in the EEG. However, there are other types of spike and wave (see Table 4.5). They may have a faster or slower repetition rate than is seen in petit mal, and there may be focal features as well. Spike and wave can occur as a result of a focal lesion often frontally located, and this disorder is called 'secondary bilateral synchrony'.

Reflex epilepsy

In most instances seizures occur at any time of the day or

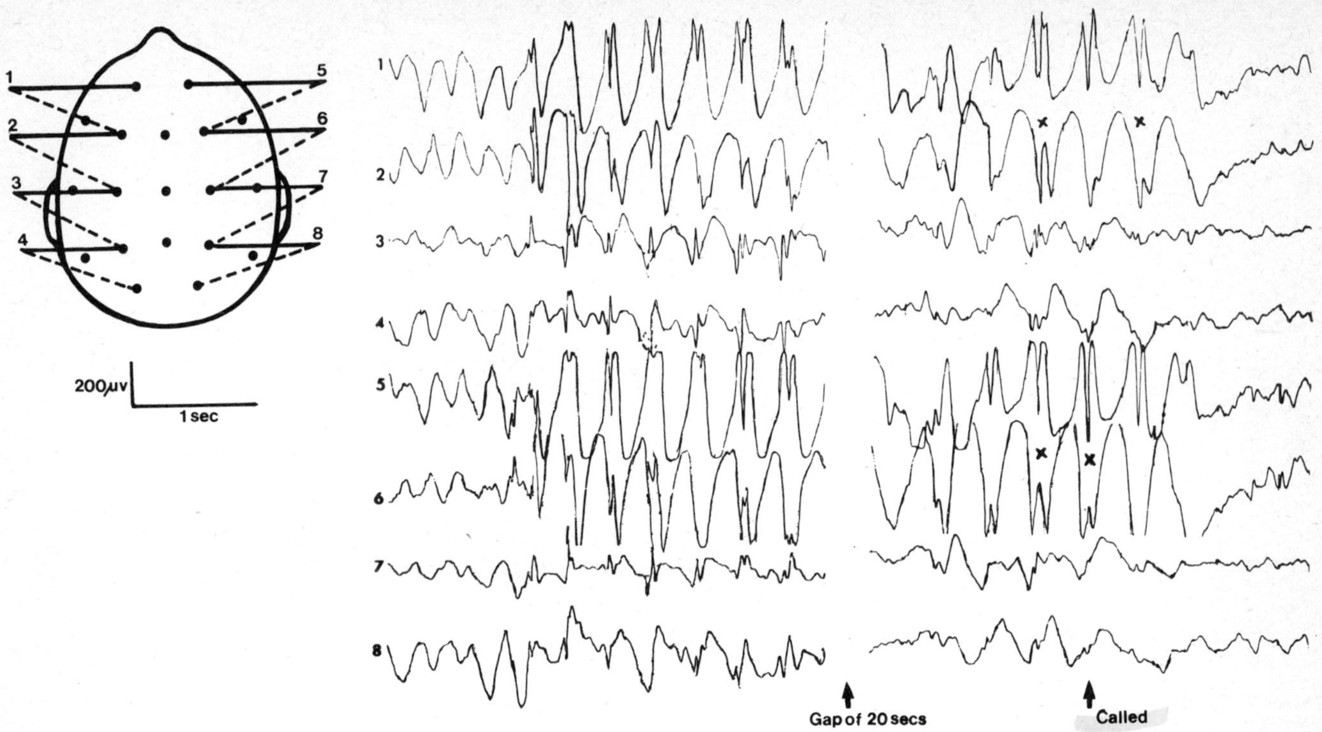

Figure 4.4 A petit mal attack in a four-year old. It was accompanied by eyelid flutter and was provoked by overbreathing. Note the high voltage – gain ¼ of normal. See also phase reversals between sharp waves marked with X, These discharges are referrable to the superior frontal electrodes on both sides. Calling the patient brought the attack to an end

night and, there is no accounting for why they should happen at a particular moment. However, there is a small group of patients who say that there are certain circumstances which lead to a seizure or that they are able by various means to prevent an attack happening when they feel the warning signs.

What are these trigger factors for an epileptic attack? They are numerous, including rubbing a particular part of the face, hearing music, reading, viewing objects, or even looking at a safety pin. However, much the commonest type of reflex epilepsy is that induced by light. This possible sensitivity is tested as part of the routine EEG recording. The stroboscope is used; it produces brief bright flashes of light, the repetition rate of which can be controlled by the turn of a dial. In a normal individual a localised response appears only over the occipital region, but in some patients with idiopathic epilepsy the EEG shows generalised atypical spike and wave activity. If the stimulation is continued, a major fit may occur. This disturbance is called 'photosensitivity' and is seen particularly in patients who have seizures in front of the television set (see Fig. 4.5). The relative may say that the television picture became unsteady and the patient went to adjust it and 'then it suddenly happened' – so suddenly, in fact, that it is often thought that the patient has had an electric shock. Interestingly, Jeavons and Harding (1970) have found that if susceptible people approach the set with one eye covered by their hand then the EEG discharge and fits can be prevented.

The importance of light has become ingrained in the history of epilepsy. It is alleged that slaves were tested by asking them to look at the rotating potter's wheel in the sunlight to find out if they were epileptic or not. Another more modern piece of mythology relates to driving along a road with a line of poplar trees on either side; the sunlight slanting between the trunks of the trees is said to produce epileptic seizures. Jeavons and colleagues (1971) tried to find patients in whom this had really occurred by asking colleagues. There was only one possible and one doubtful case. They actually put the situation to test in the laboratory. The flashing sunlight was imitated by placing the stroboscope

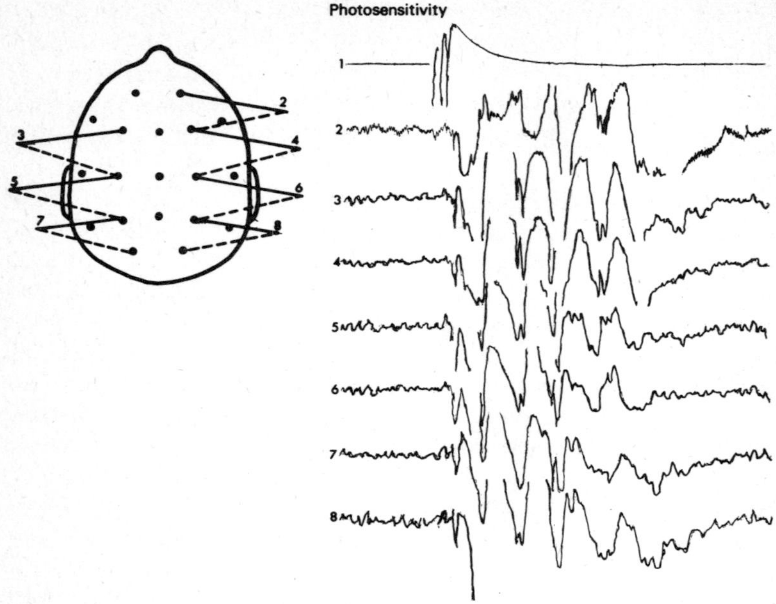

Figure 4.5 This shows 'photosensitivity'. Channel 1 monitors the flash. As a result of three flashes a discharge lasting two seconds occurred. It was generalised and consisted of spikes followed by slow components. Some such discharges last many seconds and if the flash is repeated a seizure may result

at the side rather than directly in front of the patient. They found that it did not provoke any EEG abnormality. In fact the spike and wave discharge was maximal with both eyes stimulated with the stroboscope immediately in front. A patterned stimulus was even more effective in producing a discharge.

One other aspect of photic stimulation in epilepsy concerns mentally subnormal children who apparently elicit seizures to produce pleasurable sensation by waving their fingers wide apart in front of their eyes while looking at the sun. However, Ames (1974) has observed that at the same time as these patients do this they stroke their cheek with their thumb. Hence it appears that there is a combination of both visual and sensory stimuli needed to produce EEG abnormality and fits, or perhaps these actions are all part of the seizure. Patients who are 'photosensitive' almost invariably fall into the group of patients labelled 'Idiopathic'. Other varieties of reflex epilepsy mentioned like musicogenic epilepsy, are associated with temporal lobe disturbance (Critchley and Scott 1976).

Difficult questions

There are two recurring questions asked of the encephalographer in relation to epilepsy. How often is the EEG normal in the patient with epilepsy? How often are inter-ictal features, such as sharp waves, seen in normal people?

Taking the first question, it is rare for the EEG to be completely normal in an epileptic patient. There may only be what I have described as 'soft' inter-ictal signs, though in patients with infrequent generalised seizures a routine EEG may be almost normal in one third of cases. Here, by 'infrequent' I mean fits of the order of one every six months of even fewer. A normal EEG is rare in patients with temporal lobe epilepsy, though sleep and other types of record may sometimes be needed to show changes. Indeed some would say that the diagnosis cannot be made without EEG evidence in support. A colleague once said that a single sharp wave made the diagnosis of temporal lobe epilepsy (Margerison and Corsellis 1966). This is an extreme view perhaps, but it makes the point forcefully. We shall return later to what further EEG investigations are appropriate in patients without definite features and when they should be carried out.

Now for the second and more difficult question. How frequently in normal people are sharp waves and other definite inter-ictal signs seen? The simple answer is 'very rarely'. There is a detailed study by Zivin and Marsan (1968) which throws light on this matter. They found that in a group of over 6,000 patients without epilepsy who had a variety of neurological and other disorders only just over 2% (142) had definite inter-ictal changes such as sharp waves. Further, and surprisingly, of these 20% developed epileptic attacks within a month after the EEG had been recorded. It would seem likely that epileptic changes are even rarer in a group of people without neurological or other disorders than the figure found by Zivin and Marsan. In addition, the occurrence of clinical epilepsy after 'epileptiform' features had been noted suggested that the EEG could have another use: for example, to predict whether epilepsy will occur in an individual patient following a cerebral insult, a point to which we shall return later in Chapter 7.

The expected EEG result

It is important to appreciate the expected result of an EEG; for example, on the initial referral of an outpatient (Table 4.6). If the patient has grand mal seizures and these are frequent, the EEGs of the vast majority will show definite

Table 4.6 Expected result of EEG investigation in various forms of epilepsy
(Medication is a modifying factor)

Grand mal epilepsy frequent	Positive in vast majority
ditto infrequent	30–50% negative
Petit mal	Usually positive
Television epilepsy	Usually positive
Jacksonian seizures	May be negative
Temporal lobe epilepsy	Rarely negative
Post-traumatic epilepsy	May be negative

inter-ictal EEG abnormalities. However, if the attacks are infrequent, for example only one every two or three months, then the EEG may show only very minor changes in up to a half of instances. On the other hand, with petit mal epilepsy the EEG is almost invariably positive, and the same is true of patients with television epilepsy. Here the tracing during photic stimulation is almost always markedly abnormal with showers of spikes and sharp components. Patients with Jacksonian seizures and those with post-traumatic epilepsy sometimes show no very definite changes. Temporal lobe epilepsy presents a rather different problem, and some would say that in the absence of EEG abnormality the diagnosis is suspect (Currie *et al.* 1971). However, on an initial outpatient referral one would expect, if the diagnosis seems highly likely, the vast majority of EEGs to show definite abnormality.

In order to check some of these statements I recently carried out a study to determine the proportion of positive EEGs in 200 consecutive patients referred for an initial tracing, either with a definite diagnosis of epilepsy or with '? epilepsy'. 'Positive', for the purpose of this investigation, meant the presence of clear-cut inter-ictal EEG signs of the type already described. Of those with the definite clinical diagnosis, positive EEG findings occured in 66%. In those who were labelled '? epilepsy' the figure was only 15%.

When only temporal lobe epilepsy was considered, 80% of the patients who were thus labelled showed definite EEG signs, but when the diagnosis was queried only 20% showed convincing abnormality.

Thus, a high proportion of patients with a definite epileptic history had confirmatory EEG findings, and in those no further diagnostic EEG investigations would be considered necessary, unless there was a suggestion of an underlying expanding lesion or the patient was being considered for surgery (see below). In a patient who has an indefinite history but positive EEG findings there would seem to be no further need for other EEGs (Table 4.7). On the other hand, in patients who have an indefinite history

Table 4.7 When is further diagnostic EEG investigation indicated ?

History definite	EEG positive	Nil further
History definite	EEG doubtful or negative	Consider further EEGs
History indefinite	EEG positive	Nil further
History indefinite	EEG doubtful or negative	Review from clinical standpoint then repeat routine and consider sleep record

Types of investigation include:
- Sleep – oral barbiturate or intravenous thiopentone or methohexitone
- Sphenoidal leads with thiopentone
- Others where surgery is under consideration

and doubtful EEG tracings further records would clearly be called for. The most useful technique is to obtain a sleep recording – either spontaneous sleep if this is possible or sleep following the administration of oral barbiturate. In patients, particularly those with focal epilepsy, drowsiness and sleep lead to the appearance of abnormality. If this technique is ineffective, intravenous methohexitone, has been given with successful activation of EEG abnormality, in some patients. Another technique involves the use of sphenoidal leads. These are of particular importance in patients under investigation for temporal lobectomy, and the actual methods will be described below. The leads record from parts of the cortex which are relatively inaccessible to scalp electrodes. Usually sleep is induced in these patients with intravenous thiopentone.

Sometimes one finds patients with a diagnosis of epilepsy or suspected epilepsy in whom EEGs have been carried out on several occasions, and in each the findings are equivocal. In such instances it is usually worth considering a new approach. As well as the techniques already mentioned, there are several lines of investigation which are open. If the patient is already receiving anticonvulsant drugs, these can be withdrawn and other tracings carried out either in the alert or in the sleeping state. Further, if there seems a real necessity to obtain positive EEG confirmation of the diagnosis of epilepsy, other 'activating agents' can be used. These include the injection of chlorpromazine or tetrazol; an alternative approach recently adopted in some laboratories is sleep deprivation. The patient is kept awake all night before the EEG and this appears to be effective in inducing EEG abnormality in previously dubious instances.

One particular group of patients in whom serial EEGs are of great importance are those who have been labelled 'late onset epilepsy'. In these particularly where there are focal components to the fits and a suggestion therefore of local abnormality in the cortex, repeat recordings at six-monthly intervals may be helpful. Abnormality may appear and increase, and suggest an appropriate time for the clinician to use or repeat other investigatory procedures.

Status epilepticus

Convulsive major status epilepticus, is of course a medical emergency. It always requires urgent treatment and still carries a definite mortality (Rowan and Scott 1970). Nowadays the treatment is usually in the first instance by intravenous diazepam. Quite often the EEG is not carried out in the initial stages because there are frequent seizures and the accompanying muscle artefact may render the tracing completely uninterpretable. However, the EEG can be useful in monitoring therapy. After intravenous diazepam has been given or intramuscular anticonvulsants commenced, the EEG will show whether there are periods in which organised runs of spike or sharp waves occur. These are often seen in patients after an episode of status and may indicate that an increased anticonvulsant dosage is required.

There is another and less common circumstance in which the EEG is needed: namely, in patients whose status has failed to respond to conventional medication and who require to be anaesthetised, to be curarized and to have assisted ventilation. Here, monitoring by EEG, to check for the presence of organised runs of spike and sharp waves, is essential. If the 'seizure discharges' have subsided then the anaesthetic can be slowly withdrawn.

The EEG also has a place later when the seizures have been controlled. Then it can be helpful in showing up an underlying lesion. In patients who are slow to regain consciousness the EEG may also be of value, because it may indicate whether cerebral hypoxia has occurred and how severe it is (see Chapter 11). Petit mal status is a rare condition, and although petit mal attacks themselves are commonest in school children this form of status may be the first manifestation of the disorder in young adults. A few cases have even been found in middle-aged patients who have never had epilepsy before and present with an acute confusional state (Schwartz and Scott 1971). Sometimes patients may appear to be mentally retarded, and when the EEG is performed it is found to contain nothing but spike and wave discharges, usually of the 'slow' variety (Table 4.4). Then anticonvulsant treatment may be successful in improving the mental state.

Psycho-motor status occurs, and on clinical grounds it is difficult to distinguish from petit mal status. However, the EEG is helpful because it shows temporal disturbance and not generalised spike and wave. A final problem in this group is epilepsia partialis continuans. In the EEG there is usually focal spiking over the motor area contralateral to the jerking limb. Sometimes the EEG may not show spikes, and then it is useful to apply extra electrodes between the conventionally spaced ones, which are usually 3¾ to 4 centimetres apart.

Anticonvulsant intoxication

A well-recognised EEG sequence occurs with increasing drug intoxication. The most obvious initial feature is the appearance of excessive beta activity. Then this diminishes somewhat as the background rhythms slow into the low end of the alpha range and into the upper theta band. This rhythmic activity is rather persistent throughout the record and is unresponsive to eye opening. Bursts of generalised delta activity with frontal emphasis also occur. Sometimes, a post-ictal recording has some of these features, but usually on the basis of the EEG morphology one can distinguish between the two conditions. A helpful point here is the fact that post-ictal slow activity is usually attenuated when the eyes are opened.

With increasing availability of blood level assessments of anticonvulsants, physicians are becoming more aware not only of the fact that the patients may not take the medication regularly, but also of a small group who gradually suffer an accumulation of drug in the body. These may present a picture of marked behavioural retardation (Prensky *et al.* 1971). The EEG may be helpful in the diagnosis of such patients if they have previously had a series of recordings which show a progressive slowing of background frequencies.

Will epilepsy occur?

It is well recognised that a variety of brain lesions, including head injuries (see Chapter 6), may subsequently lead to epilepsy. On the whole the EEG has not been regarded as helpful in predicting which patients will develop epilepsy, although there was a suggestion from the study of Zivin and Marsan (1968) that it might prove possible. Obviously if this was the case it would be worth carrying out serial EEGs on patients who have had severe head injuries, instituting anticonvulsant therapy at the first sign of 'epileptic' change in the EEG. From the study of Legg *et al.* (1973) on cerebral abscess, there did appear to be a helpful predictive sign: the presence of localised complexes of sharp and slow activity. In patients who showed this, all subsequently developed epilepsy. The presence of spikes and sharp waves themselves appears to be of no predictive value in the individual case since they are such a common occurrence, though as a group the patients who developed epilepsy had more sharp waves and spikes (see also Chapter 7).

Surgical treatment of epilepsy

The surgical treatment of epilepsy is almost as ancient as man himself: the results of trephining to allow escape of evil spirits can be seen in the skulls of primitive man. But it was not until 1886 that a significant step forward was made. In that year Sir Victor Horsley operated on a patient in the presence of Hughlings Jackson, himself an important figure in the history of epilepsy. Jackson pointed out, before the discovery of electroencephalography, that 'epilepsy is the name for an occasional sudden excessive rapid and local discharge of the grey matter'. The young man operated on had had focal seizures since the age of 15 resulting from a compound fracture of the skull. The scar was removed and the fits ceased. The next stage in the development of the surgery of epilepsy was reached in the late 1920s when the Canadian neurosurgeon Wilder Penfield began his classical studies in this area.

To the electroencephalographer the surgery of epilepsy is of considerable interest: first, because the selection of patients demands intensive pre-operative EEG studies; secondly, because it offers us the opportunity of recording directly from the surface of the brain – the electrocorticogram, ECoG for short – as well as the chance to test the effects of cortical stimulation. Two other points must be emphasised: it is a relatively infrequent treatment for epilepsy, and choice of patients is all important. The main criterion is drug resistant epilepsy. How frequent must the fits occur to warrant the term 'resistant'? This is debatable and depends very much on the individual patient, but in most instances at least one attack a week would be regarded as sufficient to merit consideration for surgery.

There is a variety of surgical procedures and these have recently been reviewed by Wilson (1973); the main points about them are listed in Table 4.8. For practical purposes, and in terms of numbers, temporal-lobectomy is the main procedure undertaken. Obviously selection of patients requires not only detailed clinical and social assessment but also neuro-radiology, isotope brain-scanning and psychological investigations. All of these can be helpful in indicating the sides and site of the 'lesion'. Above all, detailed electroencephalographic investigation is required to determine that the seizure starts in a localised fashion, for instance, in one temporal lobe. The first step is to review the seizure pattern and previous EEGs. Sometimes, if a focus has been present for many years in one temporal lobe, another develops on the opposite side, the mirror focus. The presence of this, or the occurrence of generalised discharge of a typical spike and wave type without any evidence of a focal start to the discharge, are both contra-indications to surgery. The ideal case is one in which a unilateral focus is found in the non-dominant hemisphere.

Table 4.8 Surgical treatment of epilepsy (Main indication intractable seizures)

Ablations	Temporal lobectomy	Commonest operation with highest 'success' rate
	Other lobectomies	(e.g. frontal). Less common and probably less effective
	Local cortical excision	e.g. following penetrating head injury
	Hemispherectomy	In infantile hemiplegia, with behaviour disorder
Interruptions	Corpus callosal section	A few cases only reported but with good results
	Stereotactic lesions, esp. in fields of Forel	Recent approach, can be used for generalised epilepsy Results uncertain because of short follow up.
Stimulation	Cerebellar	Experimental, but some striking success

Assuming that an initial study of previous EEGs suggests that the patient is suitable, he is admitted to hospital where all the various investigations including EEGs can be carried out with efficiency and the results carefully collated. The minimum set would be a routine recording, a tracing with seconal-induced sleep and one with sphenoidal leads and thiopentone-induced sleep. If there is any doubt about the case, other types of recording might be undertaken, including the slow injection of leptazol under EEG control — this with a view to precipitating a fit, so that it could be observed both clinically and on the EEG. In some instances scalp recordings are equivocal. Then leashes of depth electrodes are implanted by the neuro-surgeon in suspect areas and left in for several days so that prolonged recordings can be carried out.

Sphenoidal recording

Of particular importance is sphenoidal recording (Pampiglione and Kerridge, 1956). This allows us to obtain a recording from an area of the cortex not sampled by the conventional scalp electrodes (see Chapter 15): in particular, to pick up sharp waves and other epileptic phenomena from the anterior inferior aspect of the temporal lobe. Nasopharyngeal electrodes have been employed for a similar reason, but they are less satisfactory. The sphenoidal electrodes which are sterilised by auto-claving consist of intramuscular needles through which have been threaded thin insulated silver wires. The ends which emerge from the tip of the needle have been previously bared of insulation and are bent over.

The procedure adopted is as follows: after a full set of stick-on scalp electrodes have been applied, the cheeks and front of the ears are cleansed in the usual manner before a sterile procedure is undertaken. Local anaesthetic is infiltrated and the prepared needle electrodes inserted through the mandibular notch below the zygoma. The needle is pushed inwards until the tip is about 3 to 4 centimetres deep. It then lies below the foramen ovale and eventually records directly from the under surface of the temporal lobe. The needle is withdrawn and the wire left in situ. The procedure is repeated on the opposite side. Though initially painful it leads to little continuing discomfort. In fact in some centres these wires are left in situ from 24 to 28 hours without difficulty.

The next stage is usually supervised by an anaethetist. Thiopentone is given intravenously, a 2.5% solution in 1 or 2 mls increment every 30 seconds continuing until a deep level of anaesthesia is achieved. The sphenoidal and scalp recording are continued throughout this procedure. The patients with a temporal lobe focus show frequent spikes and sharp waves arising from the anterior and inferior aspect of the lobe. Often, in addition, the fast activity which is produced by the cerebral cortex following injection of barbiturate is asymmetrical, being reduced on the side of an atrophic or an expanding temporal lobe lesion involving the cortex.

After the patient has reached a fairly deep level of anaesthesia thiopentone is discontinued, but the injection needle is left in situ so that after ten minutes or so another injection can be commenced. This is usually bemegride and is given in 5-10 mg. increments every 30 seconds or so. It has two effects: first of all, to wake the patient up, counteracting the effect of the barbiturate already given; but also an 'activating' action for epileptic discharge, so that in some patients who have previously shown no abnormality this may emerge.

The operation

If all these tests suggest that the patient is suitable, operation is undertaken. Then the electrocorticography (ECoG) is made from the exposed brain surface by special electrodes. These of course are sterilised and put in place by the neurosurgeon. Although different patterns have been used in the past, the most satisfactory consists of a plastic sheet incorporating 2 rows of 5 contact points which are about half a centimetre apart (Fig. 1.4). Usually sampling is made from different areas of the temporal lobe and adjoining exposed parts of the frontal cortex. At operation it is also possible to record from the inferior surface of the temporal lobe and from electrodes inserted into the deep structures, like the hippocampus and the uncus. It is of interest that the brain activity recorded from the brain surface itself is 3 to 5 times greater in amplitude than that seen on the scalp. Further, the location of spike discharges is more discreet than is seen from the scalp EEG. After excision, usually of the anterior part of the temporal lobe, measuring about 5 to 6 centimetres from the pole, further recordings are carried out to check whether areas of abnormality have been removed as far as possible.

The results of neurosurgery are gratifying, for in about two thirds of patients there is complete relief of seizures or just a very occasional attack. Unfortunately some patients reap only transient benefit from the procedure and in others the operation has little effect. In these cases re-operation can be considered.

From this account it can be seen that the EEG makes a significant contribution to the diagnosis of epilepsy. Of course a negative tracing, especially on an initial outpatient referral, should not be taken as excluding the diagnosis of epilepsy. It calls for review from the clinical point of view and for other types of EEG investigation. Discussion between the electroencephalographer and the clinician, in these as in other instances, can be extremely helpful. Further, though the underlying mechanisms of epilepsy still remain to be fully understood, current researches both from the neurophysiological and from the biochemical viewpoints are constantly providing new information, and the future appears promising in relation to the final unravelling of the nature of the basic disturbance.

CHAPTER FIVE

Cerebral Lesions (ii) Cerebrovascular Accidents

The EEG in cerebrovascular accidents and disease, in general, is a subject which would in my view, repay, further research. One of the main difficulties is diagnosing on clinical grounds whether the 'stroke' is caused by a haemorrhage, a thrombus or an embolus; further, whether the thrombus has occluded the internal carotid artery in the neck or in a more cephalic position. Partly because of these diagnostic difficulties, exact EEG correlations have been difficult to establish. The introduction of computer-assisted tomography of the head using the EMI scanner has made it possible to differentiate between the different types of cerebrovascular lesions (Editorial 1974) and may help us to establish corresponding EEG criteria. It will also shed light on another 'grey' area, namely the distinction between a 'stroke' and a 'tumour', which on the basis of a single EEG is often difficult. At present serial recordings are most useful in this respect since the disturbance caused by a tumour will increase as time passes and that following a cerebrovascular accident will diminish, even within two weeks.

Another general point concerns the correlation of results from isotope brain scanning and the EEG. If cerebral infarction has taken place, the EEG is abnormal in the first day or two, while the isotope brain scan is usually negative. Then a week or ten days later the main EEG abnormality will be on the wane and the isotope brain scan is positive. Thus the consideration of these results together is of value.

Cerebral haemorrhage

Let us now look at some of the EEG changes of cerebrovascular accidents in detail (Van der Drift and Magnus 1961). A large intracerebral haemorrhage leads to extensive and marked changes. Widespread, ragged, high-voltage, very slow delta activity is the most obvious feature, and if the haemorrhage is approaching the cortical surface an area of focal delta will be seen. If the cortical ribbon is disrupted an area of flattening is found. This appearance of flattening is also observed in patients with a sub-dural haematoma. The reason here is different: a collection of fluid or clot between the electrodes and the brain leads to attenuation of recorded potentials (see Chapter 6).

It is uncommon to see spikes or sharp waves in the EEG soon after a cerebral haemorrhage, as these are generally the sign of a long-standing process. However, another type of 'epileptiform' change sometimes occurs, the so-called Periodic Lateralised Epileptiform Discharges, PLEDS. These may appear in the EEG following an acute vascular lesion, per se; but they are also to be seen when there is an acute change in a pre-existing lesion, such as a glioma, a feature often associated with minor focal seizures. As PLEDS occur in, and have been a subject of recent interest in, acute encephalitis they will be discussed in Chapter 7.

The disturbance with cerebral haemorrhage (see Fig. 5.1) is clearly lateralised, but the activity over the other hemisphere may not be completely normal. Often, in the hours immediately following a cerebral haemorrhage, there is a disturbance of consciousness, and the hemisphere contralateral to the haemorrhage will show changes appropriate for the particular level of arousal; for example, alpha activity may be replaced by theta. Sometimes the unaffected side may show a perfectly normal sleep pattern, a mixture of delta and spindle activity. The other feature notable in cerebral haemorrhage patients early on is the occurrence of a 'projected' abnormality consisting of episodes of high voltage delta activity over the frontal regions similar in timing and form on the two sides. These episodes relate to a combination of factors: first, the disturbance of thalamic and upper brain stem reticular structures; secondly, the presence of raised intracranial pressure; thirdly, distortion of mid-line structures, which is seen in many of the patients with large haematomas.

Assuming the patient survives, there will be a return to normal. With the passing of the acute stage, bifrontal delta

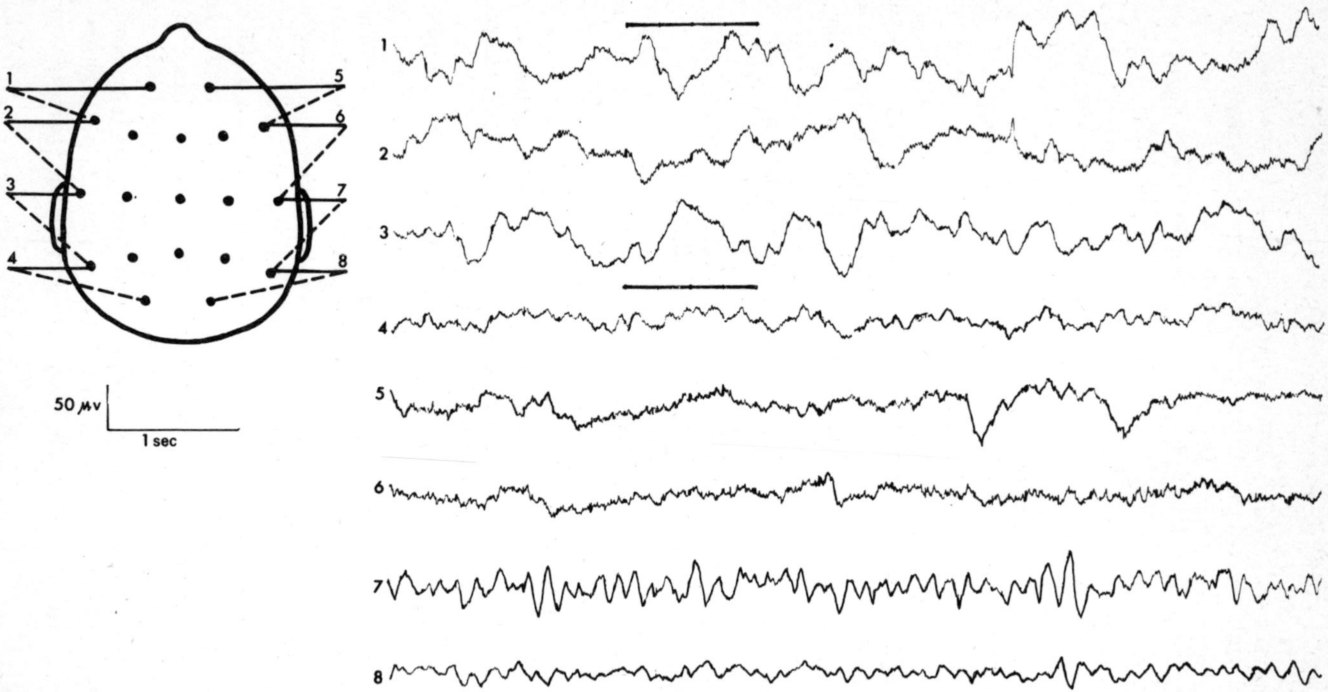
1
2
3
4
5
6
7
8
50 µv
1 sec
1
2
3
4
5
6
7
8

Figure 5.1 EEG from a 65-year-old woman with a right hemiparesis which had occurred two days before. Note large quantity of widespread continuous delta activity affecting the left temporal leads with phase reversal between channels 1 and 3 – underlined, and little alpha activity. The right side shows somewhat irregular alpha waves intermingled with some theta components. About 1 year previously this patient sustained a cerebrovascular accident in the right hemisphere and had fully recovered before the present episode

will disappear, the localised abnormality will decrease, and in the hemisphere contralateral to the haemorrhage alpha activity will return. However, there may be minor irregularities and an excess of slow activity particularly in the temporal regions, features associated with diffuse cerebrovascular disease. Months after even a severe cerebral haemorrhage the EEG over both hemispheres may return to an almost normal pattern. This obviously cannot occur if there has been an area of cortical disruption, but in some instances the EEG may be remarkably normal at follow up, though not usually in patients with persisting neurological signs.

Cerebral thrombosis

Thrombosis of the middle cerebral artery leads to extensive EEG abnormality because this artery supplies most of the convexity of the hemisphere, the area principally sampled by conventional scalp electrodes. The features in the EEG following such a thrombosis are less severe than following a haemorrhage. In the early stages moderately slow delta may be the prominent activity, but the waves may either be regular and smooth or in some instances show a triangular appearance, rather than the irregular delta characteristic of a haemorrhage. However, when the areas of infarction are small or deeply placed, there may be little EEG abnormality. In some cases, particularly during the recovery from the acute stage, there is an increase in amplitude of the alpha activity on the side of the lesion, though careful examination usually shows that this activity is slower than over the unaffected hemisphere, for example at 8 rather than 9 or 10 cycles per second. In addition, this alpha rhythm often has an irregular appearance and is little attenuated by eye opening, indicating its pathological nature.

As with cerebral haemorrhage, so with thrombosis the EEG improves with time, and it is said that 50% of patients may have an almost normal EEG six months following a cerebral thrombosis. Thrombosis of the internal carotid artery usually leads to widespread EEG changes, with large quantities of lateralised delta activity and bifrontal delta activity, as well as disturbance of alpha activity on the side of the occlusion. It is, however, not always possible on EEG grounds to differentiate these from middle cerebral thrombosis. Perhaps this is not surprising, for such a distinction is not always possible clinically and sometimes the thrombosis of this artery may be 'silent'. Tests of integrity of the cerebral circulation have been devised in patients with cerebrovascular disease, and these usually involve determining the effect of carotid compression on the EEG. This may lead to the appearance either of focal or of diffuse abnormalities over the appropriate hemisphere. However, these procedures, though recently considerably refined (Ellington *et al.* 1970), have not been widely adopted, perhaps because they may cause permanent changes.

Vascular lesions of the brain stem

Though vascular lesions of the brain stem may in some instances show remarkably little EEG abnormality (Lundervold *et al.* 1956), usually when there are lesions in this location reticular formation disturbance occurs and EEG abnormalities are seen. One interesting feature, though not diagnostic, strongly suggests such a disturbance. It consists of episodes of bifrontal delta activity which may spread even more widely over the hemispheres. The abnormality is sometimes described as 'projected' because it occurs identically over the two hemispheres and strongly suggests that there is no structural abnormality supra-tentorially. Characteristically, when the patient is stimulated either by touching or calling his name, the EEG suddenly changes from a low-voltage arythmic pattern to one showing prolonged runs of delta activity. It may go on for 10 or even 20 seconds, an abnormality that has been labelled as 'paradoxical delta response' because stimulation in normal sleep leads to the attentuation of the on-going activity or only to a transient increase in activity. There are also in brain stem vascular lesions rare instances in which patients appear deeply comatose and totally unresponsive and yet the whole of the EEG is dominated by alpha range activity. On closer inspection, however, the activity is seen to be widespread, monotonous and totally unaffected by stimuli. The pattern has been called 'alpha coma' and also occurs after head injury; in either case it carries a poor prognosis (see Chapter 6.)

Diffuse cerebrovascular disease

The question of EEG changes in diffuse cerebrovascular diseases raises the problem of ageing and the EEG. Is the EEG at 65 years of age any different from one at 45? There is still some disagreement on this question, but studies have been carried out on apparently normal subjects over 65, those with hypertension and cerebrovascular disease being carefully excluded, and for the most part the EEG deviates little from generally accepted norms for younger subjects. The sort of features that do emerge include diminution in the amount of alpha rhythm, and a tendency for it to be slightly slower. There are also some EEGs which have very little alpha at all. An increase in the amount of fast activity is sometimes noted, and scattered theta elements appear. These changes with ageing have recently been reviewed by Fenton (1974).

It is against this background that we must consider EEG referrals from patients with diffuse vascular disease or vascular disease mainly affecting the vertebro-basilar territory. The picture which is by no means specific, is generally one of disorganisation with a good deal of diffuse theta activity. In many instances brief episodes of fronto-temporal or temporo-occipital theta activity dominate the recordings. These episodes occur on both sides but more often on the left side, and some of the waves have a distinctly sharpened outline. They disappear when the eyes are open. A degree of asymmetry is often seen. If previous 'strokes' have occurred there may be some residual EEG signs, for example localised flattening or slow activity.

Transient ischaemic attacks

The differentiation between transient ischaemic attacks and epileptic fits is a problem confronting the clinician and a fairly common reason for EEG referral. In some instances the EEG can help to differentiate the two. In particular the presence of clear-cut local sharp waves would be in favour of the attacks occurring on an epileptic basis. However, in many instances we can give little help to the clinician. This is unfortunate, since a positive answer might help in deciding whether anti-coagulants are a more appropriate treatment than anticonvulsants.

Transient global amnesia

Transient global amnesia is a puzzling condition and, if the EEG is taken weeks after the episode, no abnormality may be seen. However when the EEG is recorded within a day or two of the episode (Croft *et al.* 1973), in addition to diffuse background disturbance there may be unilateral, or in some instances bilateral, temporal sharp waves.

'?Stroke' '?Tumour'

It is fairly common to be asked to distinguish a 'stroke' from a 'tumour', and even an 'abscess'. Though on the basis of a single EEG this can be difficult, there are nevertheless some EEG features which may be helpful in the differentiation (see Table 5.1 and Fig. 5.2). An abnormality consisting of delta activity in the EEG of a stroke patient may be in the form of relatively regular components. In addition there may be augmentation in amplitude of the alpha activity on the side of the lesion. Definite spikes or sharp waves are rarely seen in acute 'stroke' patients, though periodic lateralised complexes (PLEDS) with sharpened outline may occur. The main way of distinquishing between 'stroke' and tumour is by follow-up EEG. In the former there

Table 5.1 EEG features which may differentiate 'stroke' from 'tumour'

EEG Features	*'Stroke'*	*'Tumour'*
Delta abnormality	Waves may be smooth and relatively stereotyped	Irregular
Sharp waves	Absent	May be present
Alpha activity on ipsilateral side	May be augmented	Rarely augmented, except in meningiomas
Background activity on contralateral side	Disorganised, particicularly if previous 'stroke' episode	Usually normal, except where there is raised intracranial pressure
Serial recordings	Improvement	Deterioration

is deterioration, in the latter improvement, before clinical change is apparant.

Subarachnoid haemorrhage

The localisation of an aneurysm giving rise to a subarachnoid haemorrhage seems an unlikely field for EEG investigation, since neuro-radiology is so effective. Nevertheless, Margerison and colleagues (1970) looked into this and were able to derive EEG criteria for localisation of aneurysms in various sites. The approach and the method are perhaps of greater interest than the practical importance of their findings. This is because the changes they found are not specific for bleeding aneurysms, but in a particular context they have such a connotation. That is, if the electroencephalographer knows that he has the EEG of a patient who has sustained subarachnoid haemorrhage in the previous seven days, he can with some confidence indicate the source of bleeding. How was this achieved? By investigation involving a complex methodological approach. The patients studied all had angiography and EEGs. The abnormal features of the latter were noted and quantified by at least two observers totally independently of the neuro-radiological and clinical data. The two types of information were then brought together, and the EEG criteria for a ruptured aneurysm in a particular location were established.

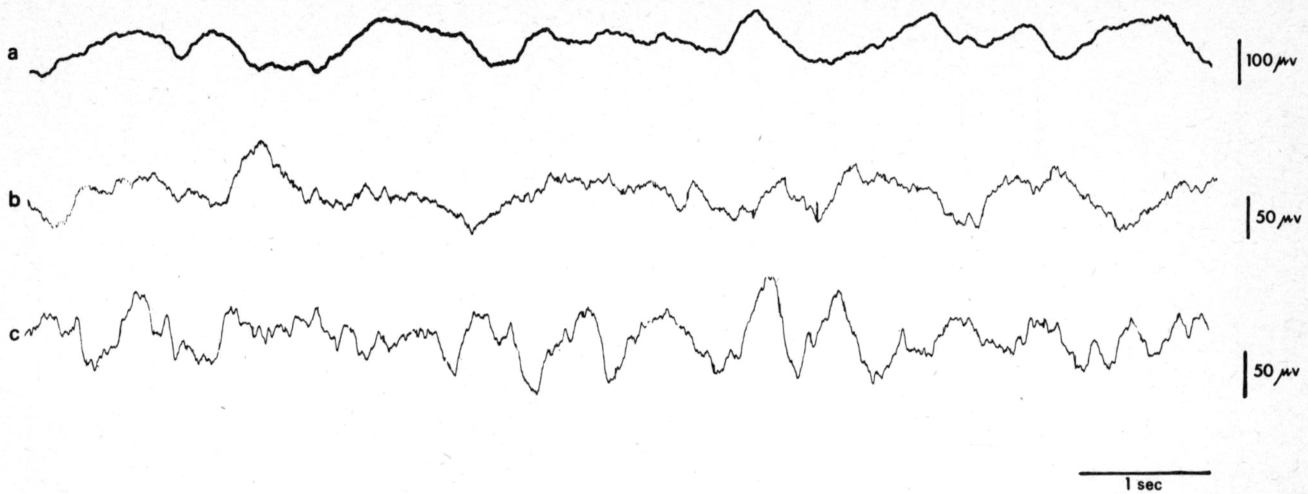

Figure 5.2 Three strips of EEG from separate patients
(a) From the frontal region in a patient with cerebral abscess. Note the very slow delta activity of high voltage with very few superimposed components
(b) From the posterior temporal region of a patient with an intracerebral glioma. Note although the delta activity is slow there are some fast elements superimposed as well as a few theta forms intermingled
(c) A section of recording from the posterior temporal region of a patient following cerebral thrombosis. Here the delta activity is less slow than in either of the two other examples and in the centre of the tracing it has a rhythmical quality

The principle of the technique is simple. First one considers the anterior and posterior communicating arteries; obviously bleeding aneurysms on these will lead to bilateral changes either at the front or at the back of the head. Then aneurysms on the anterior, middle and posterior cerebral arteries will clearly cause lateralised changes, each with differing EEG phenomena. The details of these are not important here but, for example in the case of a ruptured middle cerebral aneurysm, there is suppression of the alpha activity on the side of the bleed in association with a localised slow wave abnormality.

Certainly it seems possible to learn the various criteria set out by Margerison *et al.* (1970) and to apply them with success in perhaps three quarters of the cases. There are, however, confusing factors. The patients may be drowsy or obtunded, and this may minimise the localising EEG features. Vascular spasm and haematoma may also produce problems. Nevertheless, it is of interest that, in those patients without EEG evidence of a site of the bleeding, there is often 'negative' neuro-radiology.

In my view, the technique is most useful when applied to patients with multiple aneurysms where the neuro-radiological evidence, concerning which one has bled, is uncertain. Such cases present problems for the neurosurgeon and here we may be able to help.

Of course, an aneurysm before it has ruptured rarely leads to any EEG change, and similarly an angioma in the absence of epilepsy or haematoma may lead to little, if any, EEG disturbance.

Migraine

Migraine is a disorder characterised by transient changes in cerebral vasculature leading to paroxysmal headache. The cause of these changes, which last hours, is uncertain, though Hanington (1967) suggested that the taking of the vaso-active amine tyramine by mouth, present particularly in dairy products, was one of the factors in precipitating migraine. We have been looking at this and studying EEG abnormality. During an actual headache, EEG changes may be marked, but are relatively mild between attacks. These consist of disorganisation of background activity and episodes of fronto-temporal theta waves. The components often have a sharp outline, a pattern not unlike that seen in older subjects with diffuse cerebrovascular disease. This contrasts with the EEG in patients with tension headaches who show an excess of muscle activity but little else. Some of the EEG features seen in migraine resemble milder versions of those seen in epilepsy, and even from the clinical point of view there is an overlap between these conditions. So we have also studied a number of patients showing both disorders.

The general results of our investigations show that tyramine containing foods and other amine-rich substances, such as chocolate, do not regularly precipitate migraine, if a stringent experimental design with placebo control is used (Moffett *et al.* 1972, 1974). However, in a group of patients who said that tyramine containing foods precipitated their headaches, we were able to show EEG changes, namely augmentation of pre-existing abnormalities of the type already described, in the absence of headache (Scott *et al.* 1972). These studies show that the EEG is a sensitive indicator of cerebrovascular integrity, provided stringent methodology is used even in a condition such as migraine in which there are many subjective factors. Not only must the investigation use a placebo as well as the active substance but, in addition, the occurrence of headache following tyramine must be assessed independently of whether placebo or tyramine was given. Further, the EEG changes must be quantified without reference to which of these two test substances has been ingested. Migraine is a complex disorder and studies on it require to take all possible factors into account.

The EEG can make a substantial contribution to the investigation of cerebrovascular disease. For example, the study of ruptured aneurysms by Margerison and colleagues shows that in a carefully designed investigation positive results may emerge which are of practical value. It would seem, generalising from this to all cerebrovascular diseases, that further research into this area is likely to prove that the EEG can be of even greater value.

CHAPTER SIX

Cerebral Lesions (iii) Head Injury

Electroencephalography is of great value in the assessment of patients following head injury. Nevertheless it is complicated not only by factors related to the nature of the condition itself such as the site, severity and type of injury, but also by technical considerations. There may be difficulty in obtaining a satisfactory record because the patient is restless or confused. The state of the scalp may cause problems; for example the presence of swelling and haematoma may influence the recording obtained, and the presence of lacerations may mean that non-standard electrode placements have to be used. When there are lacerations needle electrodes are valuable since they are sterilised and can, if necessary be placed with sterile conditions when the lacerations are merely covered with dressings and the bandages have been removed.

Acute head injuries

The early EEG findings following mild head injuries are largely based on the work of Dow *et al.* (1944), who recorded EEGs in a shipyard soon after injury. In fact they studied over 200 cases within 24 hours following injury, and some patients were seen as little as 10 minutes after an accident. It appears from these studies that the EEG may show little abnormality shortly after an injury, even in the presence of retrograde amnesia. Of course, when there was impairment of consciousness the EEG was abnormal. In these studies, as in routine work, there are generally no EEGs prior to injury to form a base line. Thus, because of the variability of the norms, particularly in the younger age groups, it may not always be possible to make a categorical statement in every instance as to whether the tracing is abnormal or not. Just occasionally an epileptic patient who has a fit and sustains a head injury does have pre-existing records for comparison, but this is usually an exception. Thus the use of serial recordings following head injury is of particular value.

There are some basic types of EEG change following head injury (Table 6.1 and Fig. 6.1). It is well known that in the minutes or hours following a severe head injury the EEG may transiently be totally devoid of cerebral activity – that is isoelectric. In milder injuries, such as those seen when boxers are knocked out, relatively low-voltage records are found (Pampus and Grote 1956). So, taking these two pieces of evidence together, it is reasonable to conclude that diminution in activity is one of the basic reaction patterns. If the injury is on one side of the head, the alpha may be suppressed on the side of the injury and an asymmetrical record found. However, the situation is a little bit more complicated than this because of contra coup injury, and an entirely unilateral EEG change after head injury is uncommon. Sometimes the abnormality on the side opposite to the blow may be the more marked.

Table 6.1 Basic changes following head injury

1. *Suppression* of activity – local or general
2. *Delta* Activity – local or general, in children sharp waves as well
3. *'Flattening'* – local, due to contusion or haematoma (extradural, subdural or intracerebral)
4. *Discrepancies* between EEG and level of arousal, for example 'paradoxical delta response' or 'alpha' coma

The next basic pattern is the occurrence of slow-wave activity in the delta range. This is characteristic of most EEGs following severe head injury. If the patient is deeply unconscious, as with someone deeply asleep or anaesthetised, a delta-dominated record occurs. However, asymmetry of the delta activity and focal features would indicate that there is a particular area of local damage. Nevertheless, the more severe degrees of local injury are characterised by flattening, i.e. reduction of all activities. An area of flattening also raises another question. Could there be a subdural or extradural haematoma (see below)? These haematomas lead to decrease in voltage, because they increase the effective distance between the recording electrodes and the cortical surface. An intracerebral haematoma may also cause a not dissimilar picture.

It is obvious from the foregoing remarks that EEG

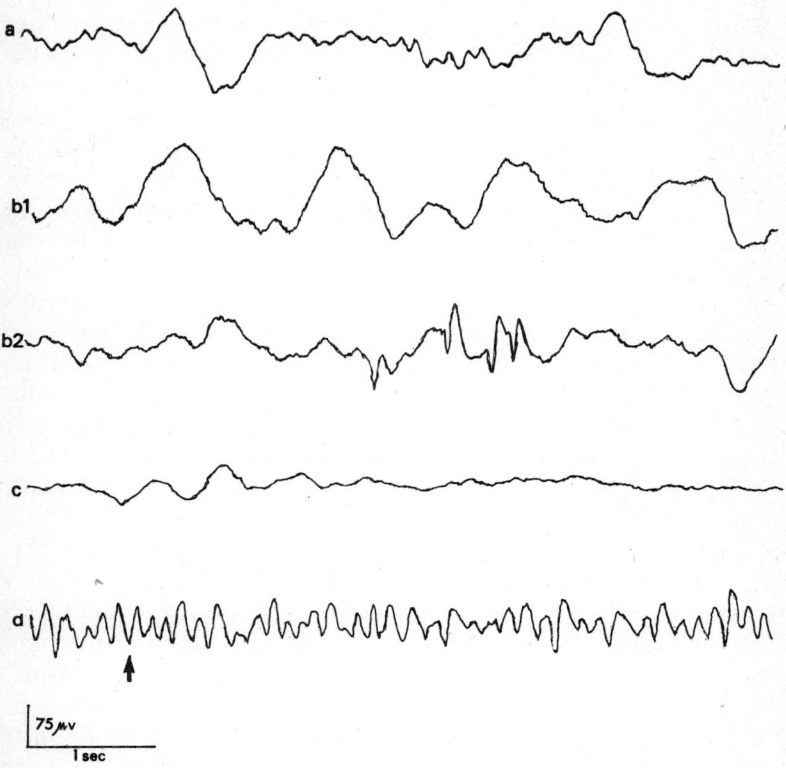

Figure 6.1 Some EEG changes following head injury
(a) Suppression of normal activity. Only small amounts of alpha can be seen separated by delta components
(b1) Delta activity which can be localised or generalised. Note that it is of high voltage
(b2) An example from a three-year-old child, with the appearance of sharp waves in the early stages following head injury
(c) Flattening. This example was from a case of cerebral contusion rather than a subdural haematoma
(d) Alpha activity seen in a generalised fashion. Note that it is unresponsive to stimulation — indicated by the arrow

interpretation in the acute severe head injury is fraught with difficulty. Just to add to the confusion, some other patterns, appear already alluded to in the context of cerebrovascular disease (Chapter 5), which are related mainly to brain stem disturbance. The comatose patient when disturbed may show long trains of high voltage rhythmic delta over both hemispheres. This is called a 'paradoxical delta response' because, in the person who is in a natural sleeping state, a quite different pattern occurs. Stimulation either causes a transient delta response, a K complex, or a marked reduction in the potentials. Another pattern is sometimes seen in unconscious patients with brain stem disturbance following head injury. Alpha frequency activity which is unresponsive to stimulation may appear, the so-called alpha coma. It is clearly an abnormal state because of the discrepancy between the patient's level of arousal and the superficially normal alpha rhythm. Sometimes beta activity or sleep spindles dominate the EEG inappropriately in patients who are deeply comatose. In most of these disturbances the prognosis is bad.

Isolated sharp waves and spikes may be seen in the early stages – the first few days – following head injury, and these do not necessarily relate to the development of epilepsy. However, there is another epileptic phenomenon which has a different import, the occurrence of 'seizure discharges'. Spikes appear locally and then 'build up' in amplitude and spread to neighbouring areas. They then gradually subside, leaving a tracing which shows very little cerebral activity in the area affected by the discharge. The whole episode lasts many seconds or even minutes. Such an appearance may be seen several times during the course of the EEG. Some of these changes are associated with minor epileptic features such as twitching of the face or a limb; others are without any clinical accompaniment and are therefore referred to as 'sub-clinical seizure discharges'. They usually indicate an area of severe damage and are quite often seen in patients who are deeply unconscious. Almost invariably such patients have had overt major seizures in addition to the localised ones. The appearance of this phenomenon indicates the continuing liability to seizures and may be a warning to the surgeon that the anticonvulsant regime needs adjustment.

Subdural haematoma

Subdural and extradural haematomas are most important complications of head injury, because they are remedial. The EEG (see Fig. 6.2) has often been regarded as an important diagnostic tool in this particular condition. The presence of flattening of all activities in a localised area, or affecting virtually a whole hemisphere, is said to be the important sign. In my view, the diagnostic role of the EEG in this condition has been greatly exaggerated, as Bickford and Klass (1966) point out: 'Unfortunately the EEG evidence indicating the occurrence of a subdural haematoma is complex and not altogether reliable.' They go on to provide criteria for indicating that this complication occurs in patients who are followed serially by EEG: first, increasing unilateral slow activity or unilateral suppression of alpha; secondly, increasing arhythmic generalised slow activity associated with bilateral loss of alpha rhythm – bilateral subdural haematomas; thirdly, the persistence or development of bifrontal delta in the presence of focal delta abnormality. The classical description of flattening is in their view only seen in a minority of cases. These comments apply both to the acute haematomas and to the more chronic ones, those which follow minor head injury presenting much later with fluctuating levels of consciousness and inconclusive neurological signs. The chronic haematoma is sometimes discovered unexpectedly on neuro-radiological examination in cases suspected of having a cerebral tumour. In these cases the EEG is rarely normal and is particularly valuable, as it usually shows a localised pattern of abnormality and indicates the need for further investigation.

Monitoring progress

Perhaps the EEG is of greatest value in head injury when it is used to monitor progress. The recovery pattern includes increasing frequency of activity and diminishing amplitude of the abnormal delta forms, which are often of very high voltage in the early stages. In addition, there is an increase in rhythmicity and general organisation of all the elements seen.

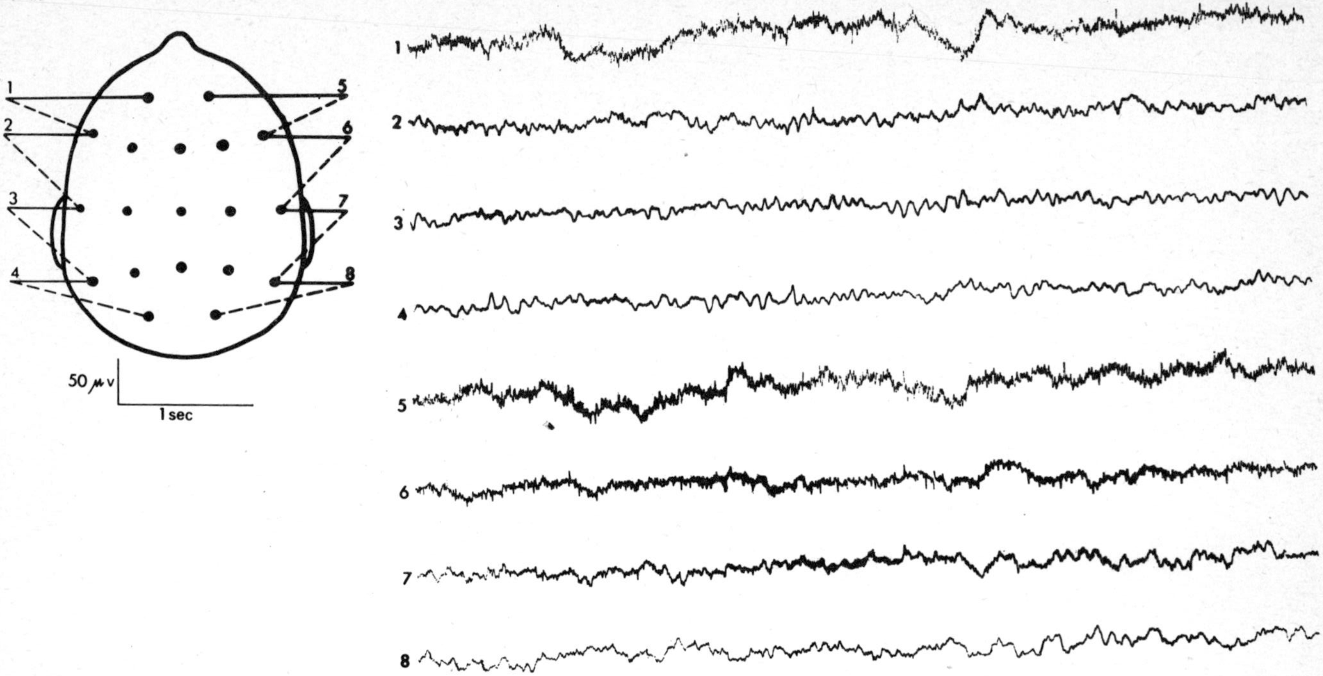

Figure 6.2 An example of an EEG in a patient with a subdural haematoma on the right side. Note that alpha is scanty on the right side and that there is rather low amplitude underlying delta activity. Compare channels 3 and 7 and note that there is little deviation from the base line in the former but in the latter there is a more or less continuous low-amplitude undulation more obvious at the end of the portion illustrated

The abnormal responses to stimulation also gradually disappear, though patients who have these may have a bad prognosis, and in any case the recovery period is prolonged. The improvement in serial EEGs following severe head injury usually goes *pari passu* with the change for the better in the clinical state. In some instances, however, the EEG change may precede the clinical improvement; in others it may give a warning that all is not well, for example that a haematoma is present.

There are two additional points which have to be considered. The first concerns the use of the EEG in the diagnosis of death. This we deal with in the wider context later (see Chapter 11). Suffice it to say here that in patients who have suffered severe head injuries and who are areflexic, requiring ventilation and drugs to maintain blood pressure, the EEG is usually totally and persistently devoid of cerebral potentials – isoelectric. The brain damage in these cases is caused by a marked increase in intracranial tension; not only the cortex, but also the brain stem vital centres are severely damaged. Here the EEG is of value but is not essential for the diagnosis of death. The situation is somewhat different in patients who have suffered primary anoxic cerebral damage, for example following cardiac arrest. In this group the EEG gives a necessary and early guide to the presence of brain damage, in particular whether it is reversible, as well as how severe the damage will be (Prior 1973).

The second point concerns the 'persistent vegetative state' so elegantly described by Jennett and Plum (1972). This has become a problem with the increase in 'intensive thereapy', and severely injured patients who previously would have died may survive because of the excellent care they receive in the early stages. A proportion of these patients do not recover fully in terms of brain function. They look around, superficially appearing to be 'normal', but they never seem to appreciate what is going on in the environment and do not appear to be 'alive' in the ordinary sense of the word. A way of predicting that this state would be the final outcome of severe injury is clearly important, not only to the medical profession but also to the family of the injured patients, who suffer greatly observing their relatives in such a state of 'suspended animation'. Jennett (1972) considers that the prediction that this will be the final outcome of severe head injury can be made fairly early by detailed clinical observation (Teasdale and Jennett 1974) whereas Prior (1973) suggests that the EEG is a useful means of early prediction of similar outcome in cases after cardiac arrest. The final results of studies in this field are awaited with interest.

Post-traumatic epilepsy

Another complication of head injury is post-traumatic epilepsy. On the whole, the prediction as to whether or not this will occur is again established on a clinical basis. Jennett *et al.* (1973) have provided a means of calculating, as time passes following injury, the chances of developing epilepsy. Generally, after severe head injury the major risk is over by the end of the second year, but the chances depend on such factors as the duration of post-traumatic amnesia and the presence of depressed fractures. These and others are taken into account in the assessment of risk. The significance of epilepsy occurring 'early' following head injury has also been assessed (Jennett 1974).

The observation of sharp waves and spikes in the EEG does not itself in the individual case indicate whether epilepsy will occur. However, in considering patients recovering from another type of lesion, the cerebral abscess, Legg *et al.* (1973) were able to establish that the appearance of organised local complexes consisting of sharp and slow activity was a clear indication that epilepsy would subsequently ensue. Judging by anecdotal reports this seems to be the case following head injury, but further research is necessary. Another matter requiring investigation is the prophylactic use of anticonvulsants after head injury. There is some evidence from animal studies that the administration of these compounds, early, within hours, following cerebral injury will prevent the development of the 'epileptic process' and thus the occurrence of post-traumatic epilepsy (Rappaport and Penry 1972). Prospective studies to test in detail this effect of anticonvulsants are in progress on head injury patients in the United States and investigations are being conducted into whether the incidence of epilepsy following certain neurosurgical operations in the U.K. can be reduced by the early and regular administration of these compounds.

Post-traumatic encephalopathy

Post-traumatic encephalopathy is one condition which is of interest, as it results from the frequent relatively minor head injuries sustained by boxers. The EEG is abnormal in these patients even before the development of the established clinical syndrome and the findings are similar to those diffuse and often asymmetrical changes seen in older patients with cerebrovascular disease (see Chapter 5.)

Medico-legal implications

EEG evidence is fairly frequently cited in court, mainly in head injury cases where there is a question of persisting brain damage or the occurrence of post-traumatic epilepsy. There are problems in the assessment of norms of cerebral activity, and in a case of head injury a pre-injury EEG is rarely available for comparison. However, the EEG generally gives a valuable guide to the presence of persisting brain damage or more specific abnormality in cases of post-traumatic epilepsy. The study of serial recordings starting in the acute stage are especially useful.

In conclusion, it can be seen that the EEG has a place from various points of view in the investigation of patients with head injury. It can provide the clinician with valuable additional information, both in the early stages and in the recovery phase.

CHAPTER SEVEN

Cerebral Lesions (iv) Infections and Encephalopathies

The EEG is useful in the diagnosis of infections of the central nervous system, particularly abscess and encephalitis, and recently there has been discussion about the specificity of EEG features in the acute encephalitis caused by the herpes simplex virus. It is a rare condition, but one of great interest, because rapid diagnosis allows treatment with anti-viral agents to be started early. In contrast, the value of the EEG in the diagnosis of cerebral abscess has been known for many years.

Cerebral abscess

A cerebral abscess is a rapidly progressive structural lesion and as such would be expected to give rise to the same basic type of abnormality as seen with some intracerebral tumours (see Fig. 5.2). In intracerebral abscess the EEG features are even more 'explosive'. Large amounts of localised irregular delta activity occur. The activity is at the low end of the delta range, and a single wave may last two seconds or more. It is also of high voltage, reaching 400–500 microvolts. The delta activity is usually focal at the electrodes nearest to the abscess when it is of large size and approaching the cortical surface. In cases where the lesion is deeper, smaller or relatively slowly expanding, the EEG abnormalities may be less striking and less circumscribed. Another feature is the 'ironed out' appearance of the EEG due to little or no other activity superimposed on the slow delta waves. Alpha and beta activity on the side of the lesion are virtually absent. As the changes are so extreme it is usually possible to distinguish the EEGs of those patients with cerebral abscess from those with cerebral tumour and 'strokes'. Marked abnormalities appear in 90 to 95% of all cases of acute supra-tentorial abscess. In those with infra-tentorial lesions the EEG, though abnormal is not usually diagnostic.

When the collection of pus is extradural or subdural, 'flattening' is a characteristic feature, because of the intervening layer of fluid between the cortex and the scalp electrodes. In these cases isolated sharp waves and spikes may be seen, as well as organised runs of these, forming a 'seizure discharge'. Some are associated with fits. Others have no clinical manifestations and are thus of the 'sub-clinical' variety as seen in some patients following severe head injuries (see Chapter 6). Sharp waves may also occur in some of those extracerebral abscess cases without evidence of clinical epilepsy.

If there are multiple intracerebral abscesses, multiple EEG foci may be delineated; for example, in cases with cyanotic congenital heart disease. But care in EEG interpretation is needed in these cases, as they often have pre-existing abnormality. The diagnosis and treatment of one abscess may lead to improvement of the EEG in one place, but a progression of the focal abnormality in another area indicates an expanding process in that site. Hence post-operative recordings may be useful. Following treatment of the abscess by aspiration and installation of antibiotic, the slow-wave activity will diminish over a period of days and in two to three weeks features may be very slight, though in some instances the local abnormality may persist for years.

There is a high incidence of epilepsy in patients following cerebral abscess, and recently the study of Legg *et al.* (1972) showed that it developed in 75% of cases with supra-tentorial abscesses. This figure, higher than the previously published series (Jooma *et al.* 1951) is probably accounted for by the longer follow-up, of up to 30 years, in the series of Legg and colleagues. There was a general relationship between the number of spikes and sharp waves and the occurrence of epilepsy. Further, there was the secondary rise in spikes and sharp waves and in the delta wave activity around the fifth year following abscess treatment at a time when clinical epilepsy tends to occur. The only predictive feature that preceded the onset of clinical epilepsy was the presence of organised local sharp and slow wave complexes.

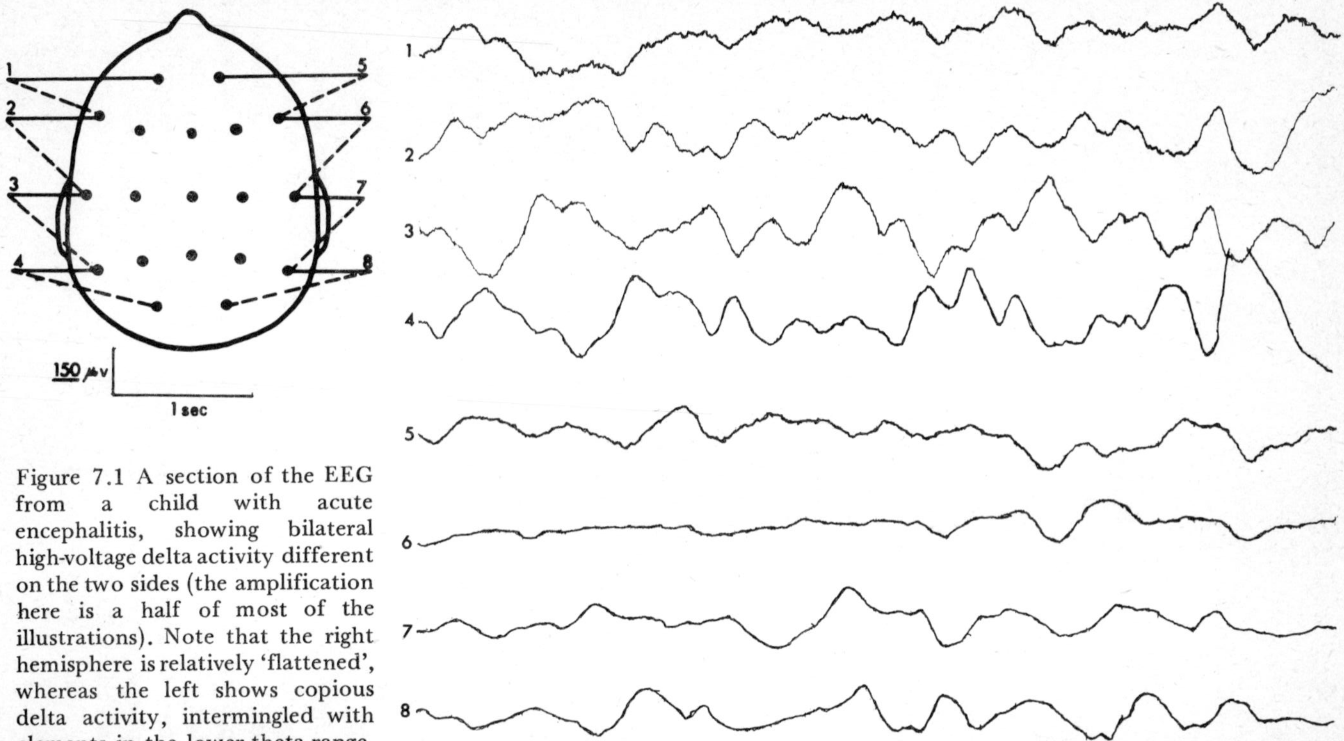

Figure 7.1 A section of the EEG from a child with acute encephalitis, showing bilateral high-voltage delta activity different on the two sides (the amplification here is a half of most of the illustrations). Note that the right hemisphere is relatively 'flattened', whereas the left shows copious delta activity, intermingled with elements in the lower theta range.

Acute meningitis

The EEGs of patients with purulent meningitis contain large quantities of delta activity. The degree of abnormality depends partly on the severity of the infection and partly on the impairment of consciousness. Usually the EEG is less abnormal than in cases of encephalitis, and bifrontal delta activity may be a feature. In the severely ill, however, the delta components are widespread and completely obliterate any other activity.

Patients with acute meningitis usually have some disturbance of consciousness and this in itself leads to changes in the EEG which bear a definite relationship to the degree of impairment in a way suggested by Engel and Romano (1959). Therefore it is not always possible to say which of the EEG features is due to this and which to the infection per se. Here serial recordings, even every day, can be helpful from the early stages, for with the beginning of antibiotic treatment generalised features tend to subside, allowing focal changes associated with localised collections of pus to become more obvious. The EEG in tuberculous meningitis is again dominated by high-voltage delta activity. However, with this condition it tends to be more organised into episodes than in purulent meningitis. These rhythmical episodes are similar in timing and form on the two sides. For both types of meningitis the EEG mirrors the clinical improvement, especially as the patient returns to a more alert state.

Acute encephalitis

The EEG patterns seen in acute encephalitis are extremely variable, depending on various factors such as the severity of the infection or a related allergic reaction, its acuteness and the state of consciousness. There may be a recording dominated by widespread high-voltage irregular slow activity (see Fig. 7.1) or a tracing in which periodic complexes occur either in a lateralised or generalised fashion, and in some instance little abnormality is seen.

The sensitivity of the EEG in virus infections was elegantly

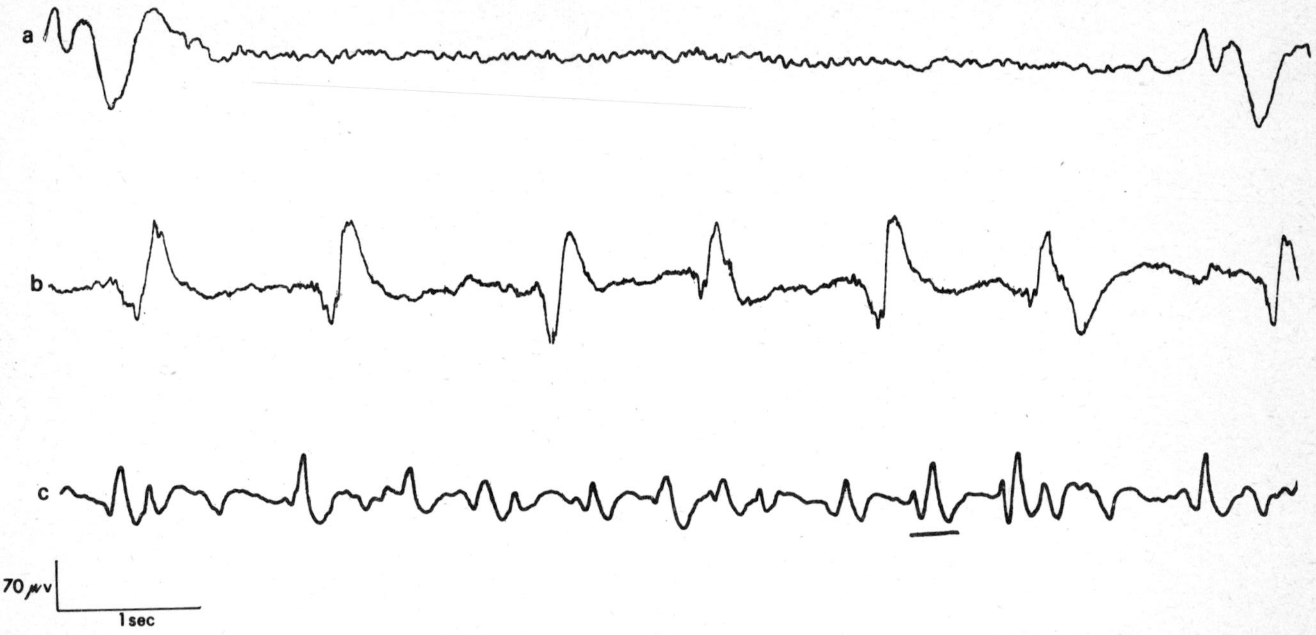
a
b
c
70 μv
1 sec

Figure 7.2 Three types of repetitive phenomena in the EEG shown in a single channel
(a) Complexes from a case of subacute sclerosing pan encephalitis. Note that the two complexes illustrated are very similar. They recurred every 8 seconds and were generalised
(b) An example of periodic lateralised epileptiform discharges (PLEDS). Here the repetition rate is much more rapid than in (a), complexes recurring about every one second, and are somewhat more variable in form. These complexes are either lateralised or seen independently on the two sides. They appear in a variety of conditions including herpes simplex encephalitis but are not in themselves specific
(c) Complexes of subacute spongiform encephalopathy. These recur usually twice a second and again can be somewhat variable. One of the more typical complexes is underlined

demonstrated by Pampiglione (1964). He, in the course of a measles epidemic, carried out EEG studies on 22 children during the incubation period of the disorder, one to four days before the appearance of the rash. The recordings showed a mild to moderate excess of slow activity; the changes were maximal on the first day of the rash and then gradually decreased over the succeeding days. These children were devoid of neurological disturbance, and there did not appear to be any direct relationship between the EEG findings and fever.

In an established case of measles encephalitis or other kinds including the post vaccinial type and that with rubella, the EEG shows much more severe changes than those described by Pampiglione during the incubation period. It is almost entirely dominated by irregular high-voltage delta activity occurring quite randomly on the two sides with loss of normal background activity. In some fulminating cases of encephalitis the EEG may be virtually devoid of cerebral activity. Generally, recovery of activity occurs gradually over a few days or weeks, but obviously in the severer cases the prognosis must be guarded. Residual abnormality includes sharp waves and spikes.

Repetitive phenomena

Repetitive phenomena occur in a wide variety of acute and subacute encephalitic processes (see Fig. 7.2). They fall into two main categories: first, those which appear in the acute cases and which are lateralised, recurring every one or two seconds; secondly, those occurring in the sub-acute encephalitis. Here the complexes are generalised, and they recur once every 4 to 10 seconds. It should be emphasised at this point that in EEG terms a diagnosis of encephalitis usually depends on the finding of independent abnormalities over the two hemispheres, either in the same EEG or in serial records, and attention must be paid to the fact that the morphology and timing of the phemonena, whether periodic or episodic, are different on the two sides.

The first type of repetitive phenomenon mentioned was described by Chatrian and colleagues (1964). They coined the term Periodic Lateralised Epileptiform Discharges and the abbreviation – PLEDS. More recently, this phenomenon has evoked considerable interest in relation to herpes simplex encephalitis (Upton and Gumpert 1970, Illis and Taylor 1972, Editorial 1972). These striking high voltage complexes recur at a fairly regular rate and appear in localised fashion (Schwartz *et al.* 1973), often over the temporal regions. The question raised is: 'Are these complexes specific for herpes simplex encephalitis?' The simple answer to this is 'no'. They have been observed in patients with acute vascular lesions, subdural haematomas and primary and secondary cerebral tumours, often appearing when a sudden clinical change occurs, such as a series of fits. Nevertheless, if these complexes are seen, it should warn us of the possibility of encephalitis when other causes for PLEDS are excluded. This is important now because with brain biopsy and immunological techniques applied to the tissue obtained, it is possible to establish the diagnosis of herpes simplex encephalitis within 24 hours of the diagnosis being suspected. Anti-viral agents can then be started early in the illness so that mortality and sequelae are reduced.

In a wider diagnostic context however, the appearance of PLEDS carries a bad prognosis because they usually indicate a serious underlying process. In our study (Schwartz *et al.* 1973), almost half the patients died, and there is a similar mortality in other reported series.

Subacute encephalitis

The EEG findings in this rare and invariably fatal condition, subacute sclerosing pan encephalitis, are among the most specific of any. When the condition, which is characterised by rapid progressive intellectual deterioration associated with widespread trunk and limb jerking, is established, the EEG shows generalised high-voltage complexes composed principally of delta components separated by periods in which there is little on-going background activity (Fig. 7.2). These complexes recur with 'clock-ticking' regularly every 5 to 10 seconds. The jerks usually correspond with the complexes. The other diagnostic feature of significance is the first-zone disturbance in the Lange colloidal gold curve. Ibrahim and Jeavons (1974) presented a detailed review of the EEG changes, indicating that in over two-thirds of their patients these findings established the diagnosis on the initial referral. However, they pointed out the variability of the complexes in some cases and the fact that they may include sharp waves or spikes. Further, they affirmed a suggestion put forward by Bayliss *et al.* (1971) that the reason for failure to establish the diagnosis on the first occasion could be due to a prolonged interval between the complexes of 15 to 20 seconds. Thus, as at the ordinary EEG paper speed one page of the recording is 10 seconds long, so the repetitive nature may not be clear. This 'catch' if borne in mind can be overcome by running the EEG paper at a much slower speed. In subacute encephalitis recordings with this and other additional measures will mean that the EEG, in virtually every case, will be characteristically abnormal.

Subacute spongiform encephalopathy

Subacute spongiform encephalopathy is a condition associated with progressive dementia in the presenium and myoclonic jerking. The EEG shows periodic phenomena but they occur with a faster repetition rate than those in the subacute encephalitis case. These are complex sharp waves which appear every half to one second (Burger *et al.* 1972) and in the established case background activity is deficient (Fig. 7.3). The condition includes a rapidly progressive form

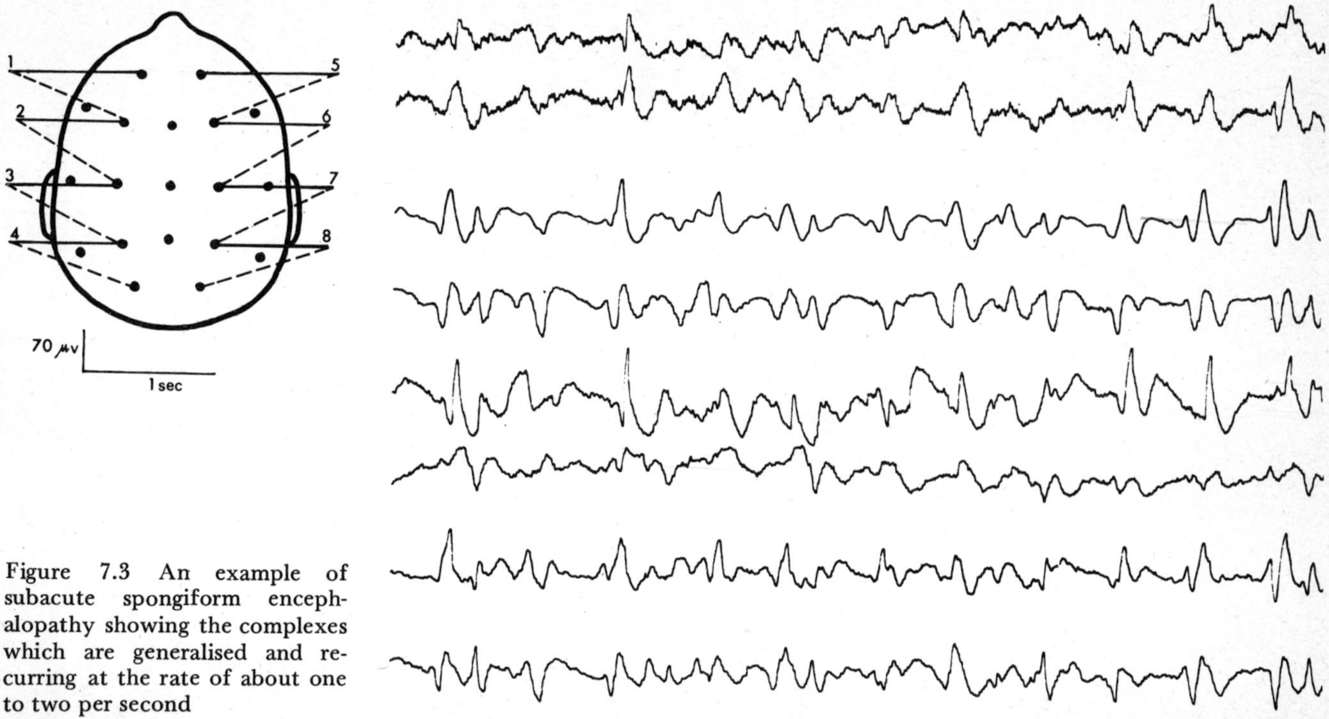

Figure 7.3 An example of subacute spongiform encephalopathy showing the complexes which are generalised and recurring at the rate of about one to two per second

described by Nevin *et al.* (1960) in which the deterioration occurs over weeks and the slightly more prolonged variety called Jakob-Creutzfeld where the dementia occurs over months. In this latter kind the EEG may not show the characteristic features early on, emphasising again the fact that the more acute the process the more likely is the EEG to be abnormal. However, in the established case of Jakob-Creutzfeld there are myoclonic jerkings and the EEG discharge corresponds with them.

Hepatic encephalopathy

Patients who are comatose with established hepatic encephalopathy characteristically have EEGs which contain triphasic waves. These were first described in liver disease by Bickford and Butt (1955) and are only seen rarely in other forms of encephalopathy such as uraemia. Basically, they can be regarded as a form of delta activity with a sharpened contour. If we draw an imaginary baseline though the wave, it shows first a rounded upward deflection, followed by a downward triangular form, which leads to a further upward rounded component (Fig. 7.4). These triphasic waves are of high voltage and maximal frontally occurring in quite prolonged episodes. They are synchronous on the two sides but in some instances show a gradient from the front to the back of the head. The differences between timing in the two areas can vary from 20 to 120 milliseconds, but the delay is usually of the order of 60 milliseconds. Just occasionally the spread can be in the opposite direction, with the occipital regions showing components of the greatest amplitude.

As hepatic encephalopathy progresses with deepening coma so the EEG diminishes in amplitude, leading eventually to an isoelectric recording in advanced cases. If therapeutic action is taken then, even in these patients complete recovery may result. Attempts have been made to link the genesis of triphasic waves to a particular biochemical disturbance. The raised blood ammonia does seem to be important, but the relationship between it and the EEG changes is by no means a precise one. This is partly because clouding of consciousness must be present in addition to the raised blood

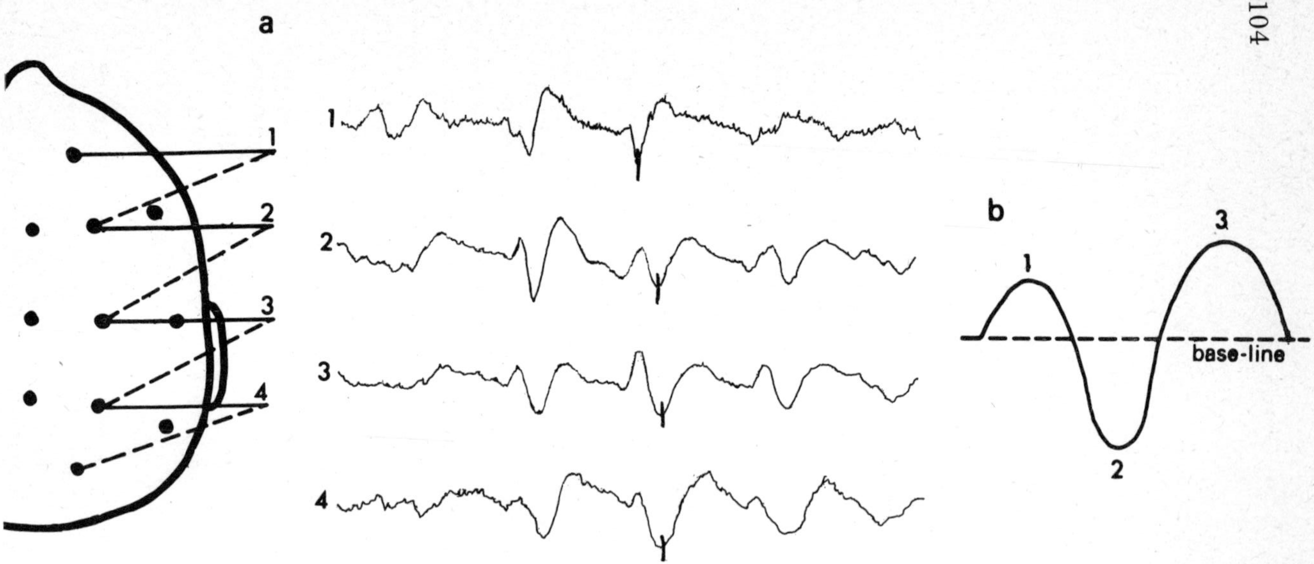

Figure 7.4 (a) A section of an EEG from a patient with hepatic encephalopathy. The complexes are generalised. Only one hemisphere is shown. Note the delay from the front to the back of the head – peak of waves indicated
(b) Shows why the waves are known as triphasic: there are three deflections from the theoretical base line, two upwards and one downwards

ammonia for triphasis waves to appear in the tracing.

One particular use of the EEG is to detect the very early stages of hepatic encephalopathy. In these cases there may be slowing of the alpha activity to the lower end of the normal range and then into the upper theta range. If the condition progresses, diffusely occurring slower theta activity is seen. With further deterioration, a delta dominant record is found in which triphasic elements appear. In patients in whom surgery for correction of portal hypertension is under consideration, the effect of changes in protein intake on the EEG have been studied. Some success has been achieved in determining suitable surgical candidates by this technique.

Other encephalopathies

Many systemic disorders are characterised by secondary diffuse changes in the brain which can be labelled as encephalopathies. One example, the EEG features associated with disturbance of serum calcium has been described in detail by Swash and Rowan (1972). This study is of particular interest not only because of its findings but also because of its methodology. The investigation commenced with a single patient who had widely fluctuating calcium levels. On the basis of EEG changes, criteria were derived which were indicative of the level of calcium, whether high, normal or low. These criteria were then applied to a series of EEGs from other patients with calcium disorders. In the majority it proved possible to predict the level of the serum calcium.

Patients with raised blood urea show abnormal EEG findings, as do patients with hypertensive encephalopathy. The changes in anoxic encephalopathy are also well recognised (see Chapter 11). While a variety of endocrine disorders are associated with EEG disturbance, there seems little point in cataloguing the various findings which are not in themselves specific. However, thyroid disease provides an illustrative example, because in the untreated patients with hyperthyroidism the alpha rhythm is at the upper end of the normal frequency range (12 - 13 cycles per second) and there is an excess of fast activity. With treatment, the alpha frequency drops into the middle of the normal range (10 cycles per second). The inverse situation is found in the EEGs of patients with thyroid deficiency.

In conclusion it can be seen that there are a wide range of EEG abnormalities associated with infective and other forms of encephalopathic process. Of particular value are changes with acute viral encephalitis and the subacute encephalitides.

CHAPTER EIGHT

Neonates and Children

Non-electroencephalographic colleagues often comment disparagingly on such phrases as 'probably within the normal limits for the age' or 'immature features seen'. They imply that the electroencephalographer is unable to make up his mind as to whether the tracing is 'normal' or 'abnormal'. This seems a curious attitude, since it has become more and more obvious that there is not just one figure for a particular biological characteristic which separates normality from abnormality: height, weight, or head circumference are given as a range for a particular age. Another example is from the 'milestones' of development. A child unable to speak at 4 years could be regarded as within normal limits for the age if in other ways his development was normal. So with the EEG there is a range, and in particular a whole series of aspects of cerebral activity have to be taken into account. It is not just the frequency of the activity but the amplitude and the distribution, as well as, for example, changes with hyperventilation.

The EEG of the premature infant

Attempts have been made to record cerebral activity in premature infants, and they have succeeded if the gestational age was 25 weeks or more. At this stage, and indeed up to 40 weeks, the activity seen in the EEG tends to be discontinuous. It is in the form of episodes, a group of waves clustered together lasting a second or more separated by periods in which the tracing is relatively 'silent' (see Fig. 8.1). The length of the bursts and the silences vary, but there is a tendency for the bursts to be longer and the silences shorter the nearer the baby is to 'the expected date of delivery'. Another feature that must be considered is the state of the

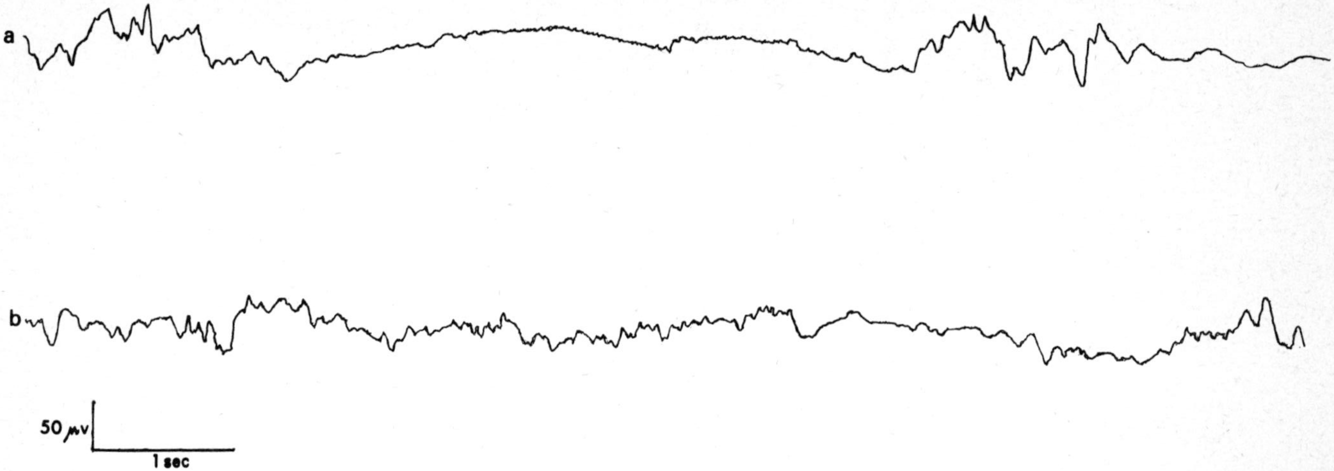

Figure 8.1 The EEGs of two neonates
(a) An arhythmic tracing with a period of several seconds in which there is little activity, abnormal for a full term infant who is awake
(b) A more continuous pattern of arhythmic activity incorporating a brief section of 'flattening' which is partial and lasting only a second towards the end of the tracing, a more 'normal' pattern than (a)

neonate. Is he alert or asleep? The discontinuous pattern, 'tracé alternant', is acceptable as normal in the sleeping baby until about 42 weeks gestational age, that is up to the age of two weeks old. Even at this age sleep may be divided into two stages, the first characterised by regular heartbeat and respiration and absence of eye and limb movement – the quiet sleep (Parmelee *et al.* 1968, and Prechtl *et al.* 1968). During this the 'tracé alternant' EEG pattern is seen. The other stage, 'active' sleep, is quite different, both in behavioural and in EEG terms. There are eye and limb movements, and heart and respiration are variable. The EEG tracings are characterised by continuous irregular activity, a stage which corresponds to the so called 'paradoxical' sleep of adults (see Chapter 10). The proportion of the 'active' to the 'inactive' is another feature which distinguishes the premature from the full-term infant (Parmelee *et al.* 1968).

Table 8.1 Some of the features to be considered in the assessment of the EEG in childhood

1. What is the child's state – alert, or asleep?
2. Is the cerebral activity continuous or discontinuous?
3. Frequency?
4. Amplitude?
5. Amount?
6. Rhythmicity?
7. Is there any regional differentiation, more activity at the back, than the front?
8. Is it the same or not on the two sides, i.e. in amplitude or timing?;
9. What is the effect of overbreathing – is it mainly a posterior, or a generalised change?

'Maturation' of the EEG

The EEG changes quite quickly over the first weeks and months of life (see Table 8.1). Activity becomes continuous, and voltage increases. However, the two hemispheres behave rather differently. Thus a run of theta activity appearing over the right frontal region may be followed a few seconds later by a similar run over the opposide side. This pattern characteristic of the babe and infant is labelled 'asynchronous', in contrast to the adult where the timing of the

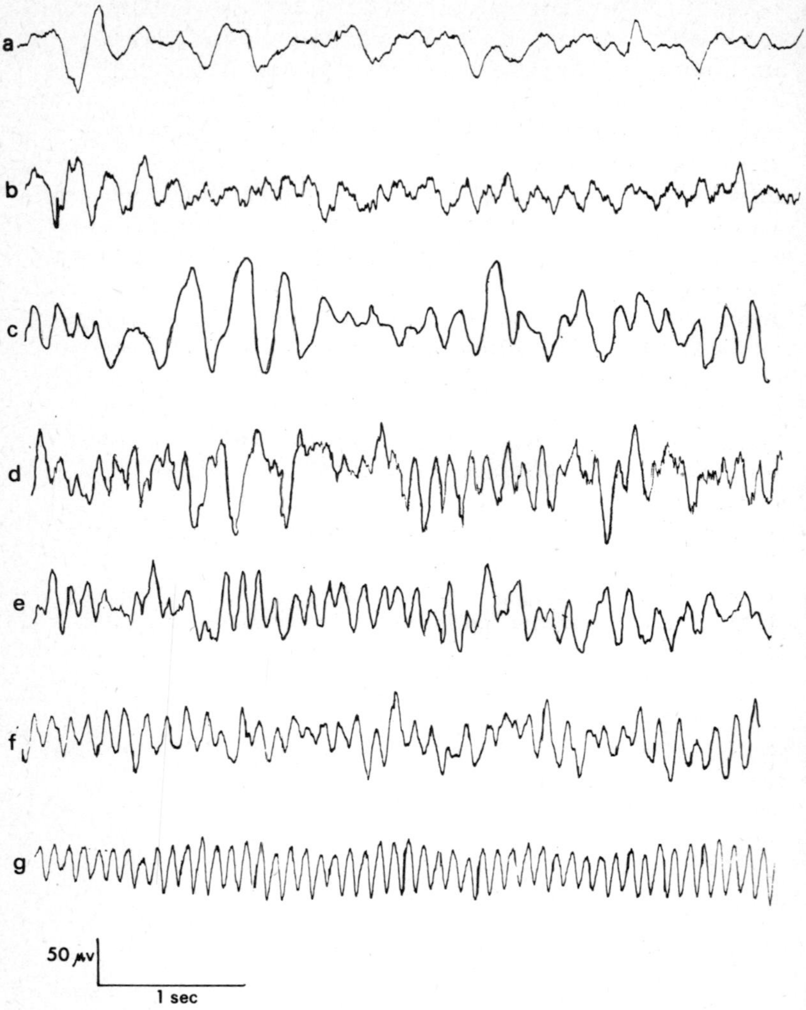

Figure 8.2 (a) is a section of EEG from a 6-month-old baby showing irregular delta components. (g) is a sample from a 15-year-old youth. This EEG is characterised by moderate-voltage, regular, well-organised alpha activity. (b) to (f) are lengths of tracing to indicate the variety of EEGs between these age limits, arranged in order to convey the principle rather than details of maturation. See in conjunction with Table 8.1

activity is very much the same for the two hemispheres. Gradually this difference between the sides diminishes in both the alert and sleeping infant though it may persist as long as 2 years after birth.

Though delta components characterise the first few weeks and months of life (Fig. 8.2), theta appears and increases in amount, so that by about 1 year it is the dominant activity, particularly in the posterior head regions, and a little alpha may be seen. The mixture of all three elements is seen widely over the hemispheres, in contrast to the adult in whom the dominant activity is at the back of the head. This regional differentiation does not appear until a year or two later. If we consider the EEG at five years, it is dominated when the eyes are closed by alpha activity over the posterior parts of the hemisphere. However, the tracing will not have the monotonous monorhythmic type of appearance seen in adults because of the intermingling of considerable quantities of theta activity and some delta components. There is a tendency for the alpha to be of slightly augmented amplitude on the right compared with the left, a feature which Churchill and Rodin (1968) have interestingly related to the position of the child's head at birth, although this view is not generally accepted.

With increasing age the alpha becomes more monorhythmic, and slower components diminish in amount. However, posterior temporal slow waves are seen into the adolescent period and are an important 'immature' feature (see Chapter 9.) The other change with age is the diminution in the amplitude of activity and in particular of the variability of amplitude which leads to the irregularity noted in the recordings of many younger individuals. At 5 or 6 years the amplitude of the alpha may be between 50 and 100 microvolts. In the usual adult tracing a value of 20 to 40 is fairly usual.

In the child, as in the adult, alterations occur in the EEG with overbreathing. The former shows a build up of delta activity with emphasis over the posterior parts of the head, while the latter shows, at least in the young adult, episodic predominently frontal delta components. Drowsiness and sleep also present some different patterns in the child compared with the adult. The rate at which the childhood type of EEG gives way to the adult varies from individual to individual, and so the norm at a particular age is often ill-defined.

It is obviously difficult in words, and even with illustrations, to indicate how the EEG varies with age. The same is true even when the whole recording is available for inspection. In particular it is difficult to assess frequency changes, and for this reason automatic methods of assessment have been undertaken. Various commercial frequency analysers are available based on the type developed many years ago at the Burden Neurological Institute in Bristol (Baldock and Walter, 1946). The principle is simple, though in practice there may be difficulties. It consists of a battery of filters, each 'tuned' for a particular frequency. One can imagine the filter as a gate with a certain width so that it will accept an alpha wave which is, say, a tenth of a second in duration but not below or above this frequency. A particular channel of EEG is fed into this battery of filters and the amount of each individual frequency found in each 10-second period is displayed as a series of histograms. Such automatic frequency analysis is useful, as measurements can be made and comparisons established either in serial EEGs of single individuals or between a whole series of subjects at a particular age. Corbin and Bickford (1955) carried out an analysis on a group of children and demonstrated that a wide range of differences emerge in terms of the dominant frequency at a single age though the EEG of an individual child was relatively stable in its main frequency component. The most dramatic change is seen in the frequency pattern when drowsiness and light sleep occur, and this is one of the difficulties in establishing the appropriate frequency for a particular age. The state of the patient must be taken strictly into account (see Chapter 10).

The EEG in pathological conditions

Because the brain is developing rapidly in the first few months of life, both the clinical and EEG pictures during these months differ markedly from those seen in older children and in adults. This is especially the case in epilepsy which will be used as the main example.

Neonatal epilepsy

Epilepsy in the neonatal period is different in both behavioural and EEG manifestations from that seen in later childhood. The seizures are fragmentary – brief shudderings or transient jerkings. The EEG often shows an exaggeration of the 'tracé alternant' pattern – bursts of activity followed by periods of no activity, the 'flattenings' are relatively long compared with bursts which contain many sharp waves and spikes. In addition, organised runs of these may be seen in one particular region; they persist for a few to many seconds and then disappear. Clinical accompaniments may be slight or absent, then the term 'sub-clinical seizure discharges' is used. This has already been mentioned, in relation to adult patients with head injury and encephalitis. This type of discharge often appears many times in the EEG with quite different locations (Harris and Tizard, 1960).

Neonatal seizures occurring in the first three days of life are usually caused by congenital abnormalities, birth trauma and hypoxia. While in seizures starting from the third day onwards the basic disorder may be metabolic, especially hypoglycaemia and hypocalcaemia (Forfar 1974). Hypoglycaemic fits however, may, occur in small-for-date babies in the first 48 hours of life. Another rare type of neonatal convulsion results from pyridoxine deficiency. It is of interest because the gross EEG abnormality in this condition may be normalised in a few minutes by injection of pyridoxine. The seizures themselves are controlled by a high oral dose of pyridoxine.

Infantile spasms

The baby who is a few months old may have a different type of epilepsy – infantile spasms. Behaviourally the child shows repetitive symmetrical jerks of the whole body. He doubles up, the head jerking forward on to the chest, as the arms are flung out in front. The attack is often accompanied by a cry

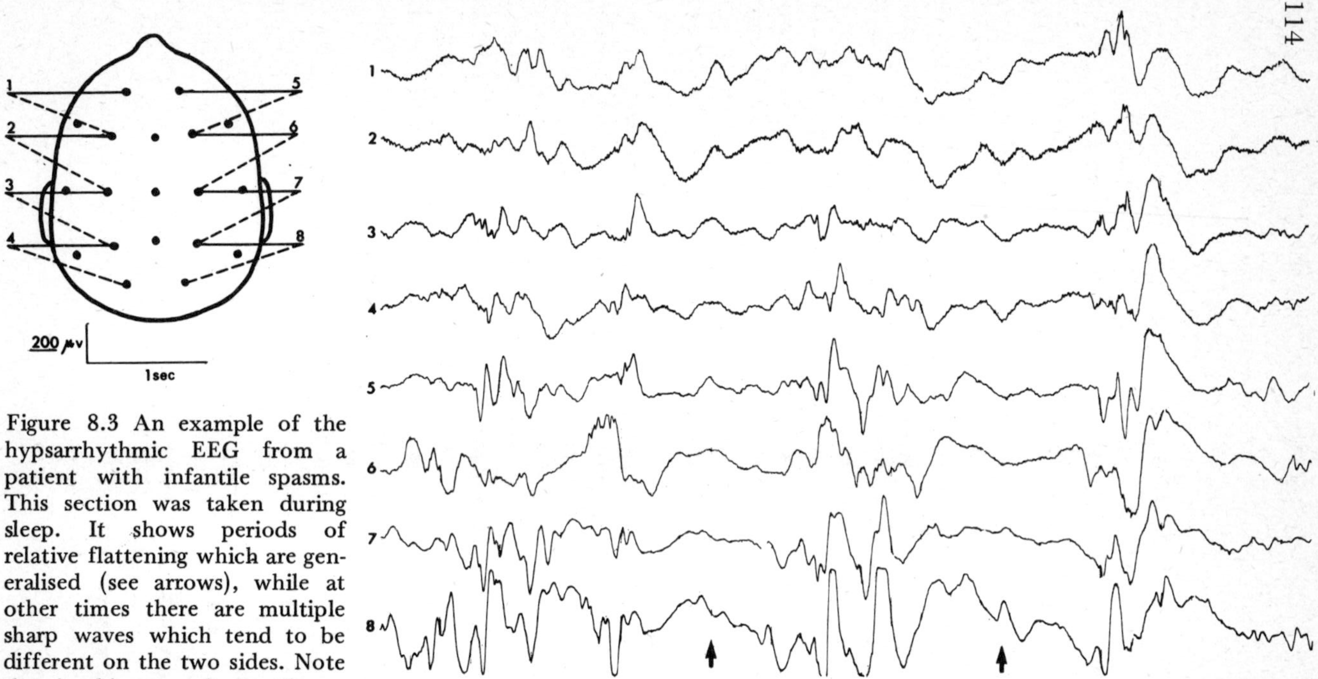

Figure 8.3 An example of the hypsarrhythmic EEG from a patient with infantile spasms. This section was taken during sleep. It shows periods of relative flattening which are generalised (see arrows), while at other times there are multiple sharp waves which tend to be different on the two sides. Note that in this example the abnormalities are somewhat asymmetrical, being more prominent on the right side than on the left

or a giggle. Many of these 'spasms' occur with only a second or two between to form a series, perhaps 50 individual spasms. The possible causes of this condition are extremely varied: birth anoxia, cerebral haemorrhage, inter-uterine infections such as toxoplasmosis, and metabolic disorders like hypoglycaemia and phenylketonuria. Over half are of unknown aetiology. The disorder is probably an expression of the immature brain, and certainly the corresponding EEG pattern 'hypsarrhythmia' first described by Gibbs and Gibbs (1952) is rarely, if ever, seen at any other age. The tracings (Fig. 8.3) show an amorphous picture of spikes, sharp waves and bursts of spike and wave occurring at very high voltage, quite randomly over the hemispheres. When the babe is asleep a different pattern is seen. Periods of discharge are followed by tracings containing virtually no activity for a second or so. The correspondence of the infantile spasms and hypsarrhythmia is particularly important, and in a young patient in whom the condition is suspected it is essential to carry out the EEG as an emergency. Why? Because evidence from various studies suggests that the early administration of ACTH or other steroids may lead to improvement in the spasms which do not respond to conventional anticonvulsant medication (Jeavons 1974). Another reason for the urgency is the fact that infantile spasms are associated with mental subnormality. Once again, there is an indication that early treatment may improve the prognosis also in this respect.

Febrile convulsions

Febrile convulsions usually occur between the ages of 6 months and 3 years. These isolated general seizures lasting a few minutes and preceded by febrile illness generally carry a good prognosis. The EEG taken within a few days of the 'ictus' will usually be within normal limits or may show only minor diffuse changes. If focal abnormality is seen in a child whose convulsion was associated with a doubtful febrile illness or relates to a prolonged convulsion lasting more than 30 minutes, or in a child who is somewhat backward mentally and physically, then one is probably not dealing with a benign febrile convulsion but with first expression of 'continuing' epilepsy on the basis of brain damage – obviously a more serious situation. There is controversy as to whether anticonvulsants should be given regularly or not. Certainly in this latter group it would seem to be necessary but some authorities would say it should be given even after a single febrile seizure. If anticonvulsants are to be given, it has been suggested that phenobarbitone is probably the drug of choice in preventing further seizures, Lennox-Buchthal (1973).

Why prevent them? Because in the view of Falconer (1974) and others they lead to temporal lobe epilepsy in later childhood or adult life. Certainly prolonged and repeated seizures or a series of seizures have been incriminated in this respect, but whether single febrile fits cause anoxia and lead to hippocampal damage which matures into a temporal lobe focus is still controversial.

Idiopathic epilepsy (see Chapter 2) of grand mal type may reveal itself in the pre-teenage years, while petit mal and myoclonic epilepsy occur characteristically in childhood. This latter is associated with brief violent shock, contractions accompanying the EEG bursts of generalised multiple spike and slow elements. There may also be photo-sensitivity, i.e. spike and slow wave discharges produced by stroboscopic stimulation during the EEG recording These and other attacks, epileptic and non epileptic, are reviewed comprehensively by Bowers (1974).

Mental subnormality

There are a large number of causes of mental subnormality. The EEGs of these patients show a higher incidence of abnormalities than children in general. The findings are by no means specific, and I do not propose to discuss the individual syndromes. However, mongolism is one that has been studied in detail by Gregoriades and Pampiglione (1966). A proportion of the young sufferers from this condition show infantile spasms and hypsarrhythmic EEGs while an older population of mongols have, in the vast majority of cases, normal recordings. Cerebral palsy is another somewhat complex condition which may lead either to spasticity or to athetosis and may be associated with fits. EEG abnormalities are more likely in the spastic group (Aird and Cohen 1950) who show fairly frequent discharges of sharp waves and other 'epileptiform abnormalities,' even if they do not have clinical epilepsy.

Infantile hemiplegia is a serious disorder on account of the sequelae, not only the severe disability in terms of locomotion but also because epilepsy, mental subnormality and behaviour disorder are frequent concomitants. The EEG is of interest since over the affected hemisphere there is very little cerebral activity and what activity does appear is of a rather degraded epileptic type. In a small proportion of these patients who have severe epilepsy and intractable behaviour problems the operation of hemispherectomy can prove of value (Wilson 1970). Epilepsy and behaviour problems are alleviated and no worsening of the hemiplegia results.

Cerebral tumours

Though there is a large variety in the types of cerebral tumour that may occur in childhood, the commonest is the medulloblastoma. It is situated in the posterior fossa, and the changes seen in this condition are not dissimilar from those observed in other infra-tentorial tumours whatever the age. The most characteristic feature is the occurrence of generalised episodes of rhythmic delta activity which appears more or less equally in amplitude and timing over the cerebral hemispheres. This activity may have a posterior predominance or be seen maximally in frontal areas, particularly in relation to raised intracranial pressure.

Degenerative disorders

Degenerative disorders of childhood are rare and present considerable problems of taxonomy. This may account for varying descriptions which have been assigned to particular conditions. From our point of view the details of the EEGs are obtainable from Pampiglione (1973) who acts as a source reference. Tay Sachs disease is a particular illustrative example. In the established case the background rhythms are degenerate, with irregular slow activity sharp waves and spikes and sometimes repetitive sharp waves followed by slow components. There is a striking response to startle.

As with other conditions so with all forms of degeneration, the speed of the process affects the degree of EEG abnormality seen.

Head injuries in childhood

Following head injury in childhood, the EEG often shows widespread high-amplitude slow-wave disturbance even when the injury itself is principally unilateral. Presumably this is related to the immaturity of the nervous system. Spikes and sharp waves may also be a feature of such cases even in the early days following cerebral insult, though rare in adults. Nevertheless, the speed of resolution of the EEG abnormality is often much more rapid than in older patients.

The battered baby

One type of head injury which is strictly part of a much wider injury syndrome occurs in the 'battered baby'. The diagnosis has both psychiatric and medico-legal implications outside the scope of our present discussion. Unfortunately in some instances these children suffer severe head injuries, and the EEG may show virtual absence of cerebral activity, whereas in others there are marked bilateral disturbances. If recovery occurs in these severe cases spike and sharp wave discharges occur in a multi-focal fashion and epilepsy is one of the clinical features. One interesting aspect of the problem was reported by Smith and Honigsberger (1973). They showed that the parents of battered babies had a high incidence of EEG abnormality of a type often associated with severe personality disorders, thus throwing light on another aspect of this increasingly recognised and intractable family problem.

The EEG changes markedly with age. In the past it has been said that the dominant frequency is one cycle per second at one year, two at two years, and so on. This view is a gross over-simplification and is quite untenable, but at least it gives a general idea of the magnitude of the alterations which occur with age. Certain disorders have characteristic and quite different clinical and EEG features in childhood. Nevertheless the same principles apply as in adults, but with the added complication that determination of normality or abnormality in terms of background activity may be difficult for the individual recording.

CHAPTER NINE

Psychiatric Disorder

There was, surprisingly, a long delay between the discovery of electrical currents recordable from the animal brain and reports of them in humans. Richard Caton was one of the first to note this phenomenon, though there is still controversy about which country really deserves the honour for this 'first'. He reported his findings in the *British Medical Journal* in 1875: 'In every brain hitherto examined, the galvanometer has indicated the existence of electrical currents.' Caton died in 1926, and at that time Berger had already begun his studies, although he did not report the discovery of the human EEG until three years later (see Gloor 1969). From that time psychiatry and electroencephalography have been inextricably intertwined, through there have been changes in their association recently.

Because Berger was a psychiatrist he was naturally interested in relating mental disorder to what was recordable from the human scalp. He was disappointed no doubt, because as a broad generalisation there is no direct relationship. Even today this still pertains, although some recent findings, which will be reported, are of interest in this respect. The other reason why psychiatry and electroencephalography are associated also stems from the fact that Berger was a psychiatrist. Many of the EEG departments set up in the 1930s were situated in mental hospitals. Now, with the wider variety of conditions that are assessed by electroencephalography, and in particular the interest in the assessment of neurological and neurosurgical patients, EEG departments have become firmly established in the general hospital setting.

Acute confusional states

The referral for EEG of patients in 'confusional' states, using this term in the widest sense, is from both physicians and surgeons. These states occur with severe infections, respiratory disorders, cardiac failure, as well as in the post-operative period. They may also be a presenting feature in their own right as, for example, when patients are brought into the casualty department having been found wandering in the street. The basic questions raised are: 'Does the patient have a cerebral lesion?' 'Is there evidence of cerebral dysfunction?', 'Is the disorder a psychiatric illness per se?'

Some patients who fall into the 'confused category' show clear-cut EEG disturbance (see Fig. 9.1). It may be in the form of focal slow-wave abnormality associated with a structural lesion; in others – those in whom the disorder is secondary to a toxic state – the EEG shows slowing of background rhythms, an excess of slow components in the theta range and quite frequently episodes of bifrontal delta activity. The patients who have psychotic illness generally show little EEG abnormality at all.

One problem has to be mentioned, the use of the words 'organic' and 'functional'. 'Organic' to the psychiatrist does not necessarily imply a lesion, merely that the patient shows disorientation, whereas for the neurologist the word implies an actual brain lesion or disturbance. By contrast, for the neurologist the word 'functional' is attached to any disorder which he believes does not have an underlying lesion. The psychiatrist uses the word 'functional' in a more precise way, applying it to the 'functional psychoses', a label including both the schizophrenic and the manic depressive disorders, while a neurologist on the whole would regard 'functional' disorders as embracing particularly the neuroses and hysteria. Hence the electroencephalographer must be very careful when he 'receives' a request form couched in these terms, particularly about the way he phrases his report.

Organic deterioration in young people

Although rare, organic deterioration can occur in school-age children and adolescents. Petit mal epilepsy (see Chapter 3) may present with deterioration in school performance, and then the EEG will usually show the characteristic generalised

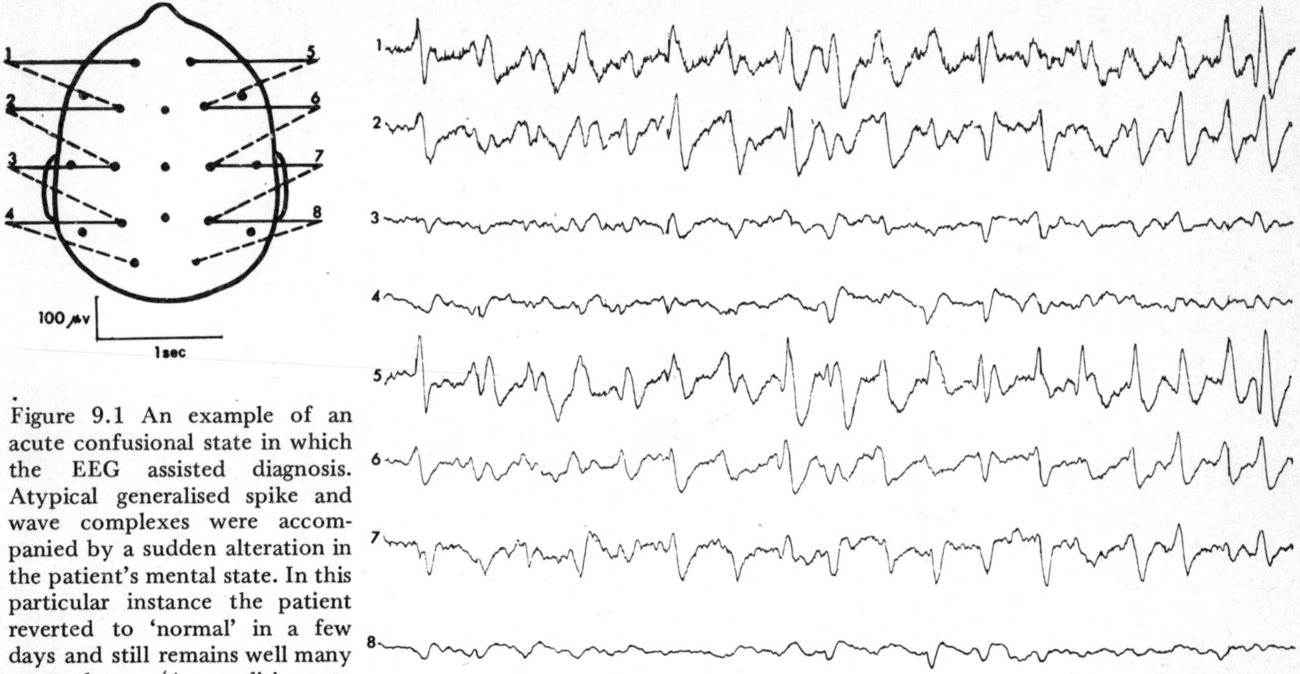

Figure 9.1 An example of an acute confusional state in which the EEG assisted diagnosis. Atypical generalised spike and wave complexes were accompanied by a sudden alteration in the patient's mental state. In this particular instance the patient reverted to 'normal' in a few days and still remains well many years later. (A condition reported by Schwartz and Scott 1972)

3-cycle-per-second bursts of spike and wave. Treatment with succinamides is usually successful in controlling the condition. Very occasionally Huntington's Chorea can occur at this age, and sometimes the EEG may be diagnostic (see below). Another condition which is seen in this age group is subacute sclerosing panencephalitis (see Chapter 8). Here the EEG is usually characterised by paroxysms of generalised slow activity recurring every 5 to 7 seconds, associated with jerking movements of the trunk and limbs. Occasionally schizophreniform psychoses occur, and they can lead to difficulty in deciding whether it is a primary psychiatric disorder or the first signs of organic disease.

Pre-senile dementias

Pre-senile dementias are a large heterogeneous category of disorders presenting before the age of 60 or 65 years, an arbitrary cut-off point. There are some conditions which are specific for the presenium while others are responsible for dementia in any age group. Cerebral tumours are one example of the latter; they may present with memory disorders, depression and other psychological and behavioural changes. The EEG findings in this condition have already been described (see Chapter 3).

Huntington's Chorea is a disorder most commonly seen in the presenium. Intellectual deterioration like the chorea itself is a cardinal feature, though this may have been preceded by anti-social behaviour. The characteristic EEG pattern of the disorder is the disappearance of alpha activity, and indeed the tracings may show little whatsoever in the way of rhythmic cerebral potentials (see Fig. 9.2). In particular the amplitude is very low, less than 10 microvolts. The phenomena usually seen during sleep are also abnormal (Sishta *et al.* 1974). If present, these findings are diagnostic, but unfortunately they are not often an early sign of the condition and are usually seen in Huntington's Chorea patients who have marked degenerative changes, of both the caudate nuclei and the frontal lobes (Scott *et al.* 1972). It will be recalled that Huntington's Chorea, which is inherited as a mendelian dominant, expresses itself in the late 30s and 40s

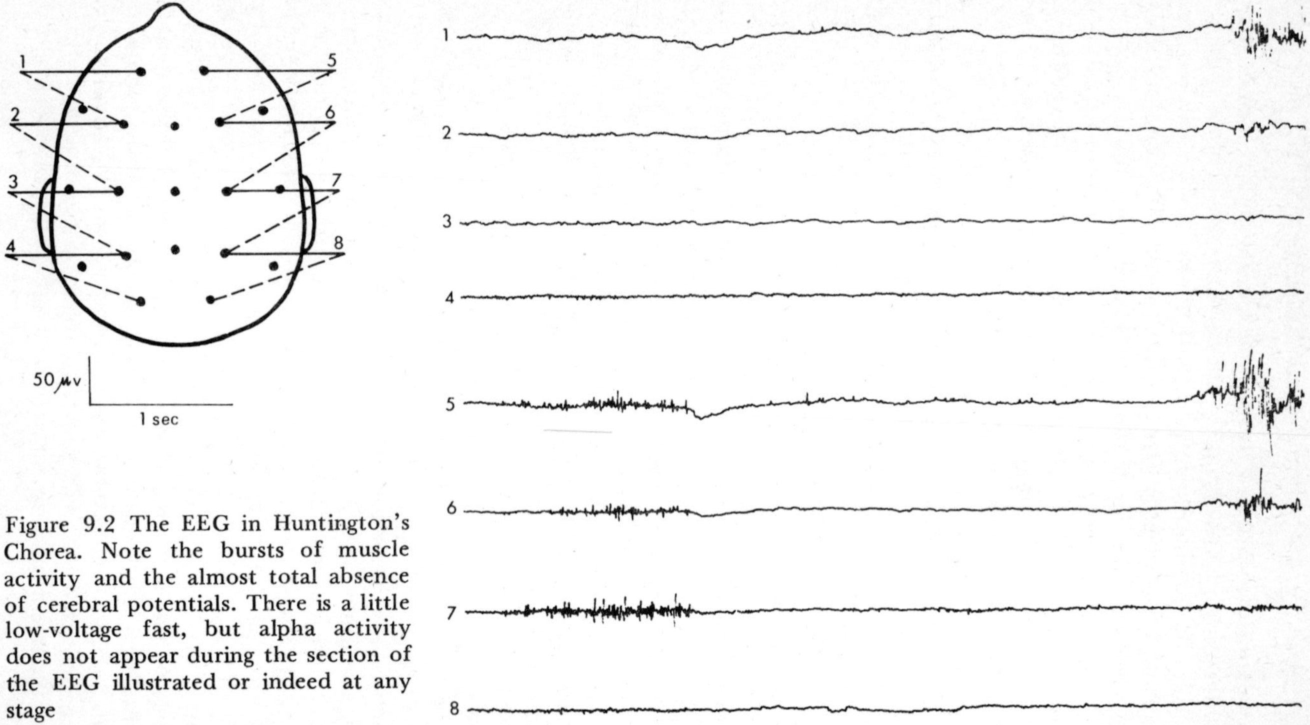

Figure 9.2 The EEG in Huntington's Chorea. Note the bursts of muscle activity and the almost total absence of cerebral potentials. There is a little low-voltage fast, but alpha activity does not appear during the section of the EEG illustrated or indeed at any stage

after the carrier has already had a family. Hence one of the problems is of course to detect carriers before the expression of the clinical disorder. Detailed EEG studies of families with Huntington's Chorea have unfortunately failed to disclose any characteristic pre-symptomatic changes.

Alzheimer's disease is a well-recognised pre-senile dementia. The EEG shows a high incidence of abnormality in this disorder (Letemandia and Pampiglione 1958), with generalised disorganisation, loss of alpha activity and intermingled theta components. More strikingly random high-voltage delta episodes occur over the frontal regions and there are scattered sharp waves. If a sleep record is carried out, the electrical activity appropriate for the various sleep stages is markedly depleted.

There are other pre-senile dementias which have well-recognised EEG patterns; for example, the subacute spongiform encephalopathy and the related Jakob-Creutzfeldt syndrome. Both are characterised by intellectual impairment. The former has a more rapid course and, although there is controversy about some aspects of the EEG, in both there is a striking abnormality with disappearance of background activity and repetitive sharp waves or complexes occurring every half to one second. This pattern is seen early in the chronic spongiform encephalopathy and probably later in Jacob-Creutzfeldt syndrome (see Chapter 7).

Senile dementias

The distinction between the pre-senile and the senile dementias is arbitary. However, the senile group contains a large number of patients who have dementia which is of vascular origin. Here general disorganisation is the most characteristic feature, with considerable differences between the hemispheres. This may relate partly to previous 'stroke' episodes. If they have occurred in the recent past there may be quite marked and definite localised abnormalities.

Considering the whole group of degenerative disorders it is important to note that the more rapid the process the more likely is it that EEG disturbance will be seen. This applies to all the disorders and may explain the lack of positive EEG findings in some on first referral. Here computerised tomography of the head using the EMI scanner may have a special place in patients who present with dementia. Although its role is not as yet established it does appear that this technique can detect increase in ventricular size without recourse to 'invasive' neuroradiological procedures, as well as the presence of focal lesions such as tumours or haematomas.

Psychiatric disorders

As has been emphasised, in psychiatric disorder, unless it has an organic basis in the terms neurologists use, the EEG may not show much disturbance. However, we must examine the different conditions in order to see what in fact there is in the recordings. Taking first the overall view of patients with psychiatric disorder, these show more abnormality than the control population; but the findings are largely non-specific. The anxious or neurotic patient may have little in the EEG apart from an excess of muscle potentials and an absence of alpha activity, perhaps related to their unusually high level of arousal. A normal person if confronted with mental arithmetic or a complex visual stimulus shows little alpha rhythm, a condition comparable with that in the anxious patient. An hysterical patient having attacks may show a normal EEG the moment the 'seizure' has ceased. This is most unusual in the epileptic patient and can be taken as evidence of a diagnosis of 'non-epilepsy' (see Chapter 4). Patients who have coma or stupor without organic basis have EEGs within normal limits (Hopkins 1973).

Personality disorders

When we consider the patients with personality disorders a new aspect emerges. Their EEGs often contain features appropriate for a younger age; that is, they show signs of 'immaturity'. Posterior temporal slow waves are the most characteristic. These appear on both sides, but usually with a right-sided predominance, and attenuate when the eyes are open. Studies on patients with violent behaviour have recently been reviewed (Fenton 1974), and it appears that the EEG is different in those in whom the behaviour was premeditated from those in whom it occurred in an impulsive fashion. This latter group exhibit 'immature' phenomena. Murderers have also been studied in a similar way and the same pattern emerges. Abnormality of sex chromosome complement also leads to EEG abnormality. This is particularly true of the patients with the XXY pattern as compared to the XYY cases (Fenton *et al.* 1971). Features include significant generalised excesses of theta activity and a slow dominant rhythm.

Psychoses

Psychoses can be separated into two main classes, the manic depressive and the schizophrenic. In neither are there very specific EEG features, and on superficial inspection of the EEG little or nothing may emerge. The manic depressive patients on the whole have the more 'normal' tracings, while the schizophrenic patients may have features reminiscent of the inter-ictal EEG of epileptic patients: for example, brief bursts of atypical spike and wave. The records are generally disorganised with an excess of slow components. Catatonic patients are particularly likely to show these phemonena, all of which are extremely uncommon in the EEGs of manic depressive patients. In patients with recurrent psychoses serial tracings have been studied, for example Gjessing *et al.* (1967), and Harding (1974) and clear-cut differences are found between the normal and psychotic state.

Visual inspection of the EEG can yield, as we shall see, a surprising amount of information, and quite often it can usefully be supplemented by employing a frequency analyser (see Chapter 8). This automatic device produces histograms of individual frequencies, so that slight shifts in the dominant rhythm can be detected with ease. In patients with manic depressive psychoses, there may be a difference of 1 cycle per second in the alpha activity when the manic and the depressive phases are compared. In an individual patient it is often possible on a careful visual inspection to determine, using this knowledge, whether the patient was elated or depressed.

In a recent study (Scott and Schwartz 1975) an extension of detailed visual analysis techniques was used. The first part of the investigation concerned a patient who had both schizophrenic and depressive episodes and then recovered, all within the space of three months. Twelve EEGs were carried out at weekly intervals during her illness. Subsequently these were masked and randomised and then given to a rater who knew only in outline about the illness. He was asked to quantify the EEG phenomena seen. Subsequently these findings were related to the patient's mental state. Certain criteria emerged, some of which typified the depressive and others the schizophrenic state. In the second part of the investigation a group of EEGs from schizophrenic and depressed patients was collected, masked and randomised and rated on the same basis. The rater was able to separate the recordings with alacrity into those characteristic of the depressive and those of the schizophrenic category, he was correct in 17 out of 21 instances. It might be thought that more exact categorisation would have been possible. However, psychiatric diagnosis itself is not particularly exact, and in any case the EEG phenomena themselves were of a relatively minor nature and might have been overlooked on more cursory inspection. This investigation proved that detailed visual examination with reduction of the subjective element produces useful additional information which can then be used during the ordinary everyday 'eyeballing' techniques.

It is hoped that, with more sophisticated methods both in terms of behavioural assessment of the patients and of computer analysis, an even more effective use of the EEG will be possible, not only for diagnosis but also for the greater understanding of the underlying neuro-physiological basis of mental disorder.

Epilepsy and mental disorder

One particular condition of interest is the schizophrenia-like psychosis of epilepsy first described in detail by Slater *et al.* (1963). Patients with this disorder show temporal lobe foci, though to display them it may be necessary to use sphenoidal leads (see Chapter 4), and thiopentone-induced sleep.

Flor-Henry (1969) noted that left-sided foci were associated with this type of schizophrenia while right-sided foci were found in patients with manic depressive psychosis and Taylor (1972) found in non-psychotic temporal lobe patients that there was a tendency for left-sided foci to be associated with antisocial behaviour and right-sided ones with neurotic symptoms.

The effects of treatment

When looking at the EEGs of psychiatric patients it is important to consider possible effects of treatment. Drugs are the most obvious example, and they have markedly varying effects on the EEG in different individuals. As a result, attempts have been made to relate changes seen to treatment response. This approach has not in my view been entirely successful. In general most psychotropic drugs lead to a decrease in the amount and frequency of alpha activity with augmentation of slower frequencies, while fast activity is not changed much. On the other hand barbiturates and benzodiazepine compounds cause a marked augmentation in the amount of fast activity and in some instances to an increase in the alpha frequency as well. Focal abnormalities are often supressed with regular oral dosage of benzodiazepines. Another feature that concerns mainly the anti-depressant drugs is the activation of 'epileptic abnormalities' in the form of sharp waves and spike and wave. These drugs may, in some individuals, lead to overt seizures, which usually occur in those who have a history of pre-existing brain disease or family history of epilepsy (Betts *et al.* 1968, Dallos and Heathfield 1969). One innovation in psychiatry has been the use of depot injections of phenothiazine drugs in schizophrenic patients. Recently we have seen two patients in a stuporose state apparently as a result of these injections. They presented without any definite history and showed in their EEGs a slow dominant frequency which did not respond to eye opening. After a certain amount of 'detective work' the history of previous psychiatric illness came to light and also the actual treatment they received.

The effects of electro-convulsive therapy (ECT) must be

taken into consideration. If the EEG is recorded during the actual treatment session the tracings are like that during a spontaneous grand mal fit; namely, generalised spikes. There is, however, the modifying factor of the anaesthetic which is almost invariably used nowadays. The overall effects of ECT in terms of EEG change are minimal, unless the patient has had prolonged and repeated courses. Just occasionally, however, a patient is seen with generalised disorganisation of background activity and the occurrence of episodic frontal delta. These changes are symmetrical, and usually they have completely disappeared within three months after the termination of a course of treatment. With the institution of unilaterial ECT the changes are somewhat different (Volavka *et al.* 1972).

The operation of pre-frontal leucotomy is now relatively rarely performed, although occasionally patients who have had this procedure in the past are referred for an EEG. If the operation has been carried out relatively recently there is generalised delta activity of high voltage and with a frontal preponderance. Another feature of patients who have had this operation is the disturbance of the electrical activity appropriate for sleep – for example, spindles which normally are over the frontal regions in stage 2 sleep are depleted. This is probably related to the extent of the lesions, in particular interruption of the fibres linking the cortex to the mid-line reticular structures. There may also be sharp waves visible over the frontal regions. The reason for referral is often the occurrence of epilepsy, and then ordinarily one would expect to see copious sharp waves, and this is almost always the case.

Mental functions

From the earliest days there has been a hope that a distinct relationship could be established between personality, intelligence, mood changes and the EEG. The first investigations performed concerned the alpha rhythm. Three 'alpha' types were described: the R type, Responsive alpha; the P type, with Persistent alpha; and the M type who showed only Minimal alpha at any time. These types were then related to the use of visual imagery by the individual, but no clear cut results emerged. Other studies have involved detailed assessment of the EEG either by eye or computer and the use of personality inventories. These also failed to establish any clear-cut relationships between for example extraversion and introversion EEG features (Fenton and Scotton 1967). Nevertheless, at the present time various types of computer analysis are in progress in an attempt to find positive association, and some are beginning to emerge. For example Fenwick *et al.* (1975), in a detailed study of schoolchildren, showed that intellectually retarded 14-year-olds were more likely to have disorganised EEGs deficient in alpha that their intellectually superior brethren – a not very stimulating result, but it augurs well for the future.

Computers have also been used in evoked response studies. These will be described later (Chapter 13), but mention of an interesting type of response from the point of view of mental functioning must be made here. This is the 'expectancy wave,' described by Grey Walter and colleagues in 1964, and now known as the Contingent Negative Variation (CNV). This is a delta wave seen widely over the scalp following a warning stimulus in a period while the subject is anticipating another stimulus which requires his action. Generally, the warning stimulus is a tone, and the next stimulus, a second or so later, is a series of flashes. The subject is required to press a button, as soon as the flashes begin, to turn them off. The 'expectancy' wave can sometimes be seen in the ordinary EEG. Usually, however, it is best examined with a computer which can summate the responses to 20 or more tone-flash combinations. The experimental conditions can be varied and tests carried out to determine what parameters affect the amplitude of the expectancy wave. More important from the clinical point of view is its application to psychiatric patients. Results are as yet incomplete, but actively hallucinating schizophrenics tend to have smaller expectancy waves than other schizophrenic patients. There is also a difference between psychopaths and normals, the former showing the smaller response (see also Chapter 13).

Just 45 years have elapsed in the study of the EEG with

relation to mental functioning and mental disorder, and we are just beginning to get a few definite results. This type of advance is to a large extent based on improvements in technology, but with the wider availability of computers in hospitals and particularly in EEG departments even greater progress can be expected in the not too distant future.

CHAPTER TEN

Sleep

Sleep is important in electroencephalography for three main reasons. First, certain types of abnormality, particularly focal epileptic discharges, are 'activated,' that is enhanced, by the change in the patient from the alert to the sleeping state. In fact, it is often in the drowsy phase that previously undisclosed abnormalities emerge. For this reason patients in whom there is doubt about the diagnosis of epilepsy or its EEG manifestations are given an oral barbiturate to promote sleep. Secondly, the EEG is used to explore the neuro-psychological basis of sleep, and it has become in this field a valuable research tool. Thirdly, the EEG can be used to test the effects of drugs and compare their actions, by determining the speed of onset and the depth of sleep achieved.

The nature of sleep

There are many mysteries surrounding sleep and consciousness; for example, the purpose of sleep, which occupies about a third of the life span, is still uncertain. What we do know indicates that, though it is a state accompanied by behavioural inactivity, it is not an inert one in terms of physiological or mental processes, a point to which we shall return later. Sleep can readily be distinguished from coma produced by diseases or drugs, for in sleep the subject can be roused, be it easily or with difficulty, depending on the depth of sleep, while this is impossible in coma. There is, however, an intermediate stage, stupor, which occurs in some forms of mental illness and certain brain lesions. A stuporose patient is incompletely responsive to stimuli and though immobile he can be surprisingly aware of what is going on around him. For example, a patient with catatonic schizophrenia may sit in the corner of the room hardly moving for weeks, and yet when he recovers he is able to recount all that happened.

Another of the mysteries concerning sleep is how we actually 'fall asleep'. This is partly related to habits. People regularly go to bed at a particular time of day. However, there is another aspect which shows itself when a long plane journey is taken resulting in a time change of 6 to 8 hours. We try to go to sleep by the local clocks. If we succeed we may still wake by the time dictated on our 'inner biological clock'. Its 24-hour cycle has a powerful hold over us, controlling not just wakefulness and sleep but many other processes, including serum electrolytes. There is even a diurnal-nocturnal variation in the frequency of alpha activity (see Chapter 2). The rhythm of the biological clock is relatively resistant to change. It has been shown by those who have subjected themselves to a neutral environment, for example, at the bottom of a cave for weeks or months, that most individuals show fairly slight shifts, either consistent lengthening or consistent shortening in the 24-hour cycle.

Exactly what significance this has in terms of mental and physiological functioning is not known, but research has demonstrated that many of the body processes have a diurnal-nocturnal rhythm, and some are directly related to certain phases of sleep only. These studies have been carried out in subjects with in-dwelling catheters through which small blood samples can repeatedly be taken without disturbing them in the night. The EEG at the time when the growth hormone secretion is greatest shows high-voltage delta activity. Growth hormone increases the rate of synthesis of protein and ribo-nucleic acid and presumably accounts for the fact that division of cells in the skin and the bone marrow take place mainly during sleep.

We thus return to the old and trite notion that sleep has a restorative function at least for physical processes. If so, then we need nourishment during sleep. This seems almost too simple to be true, but interestingly enough Oswald and colleagues (Brezinova and Oswald 1972) have shown in their sleep laboratory that a well-known and highly advertised milky beverage taken before retiring does apparently promote better sleep!

Physical processes are not restricted to the body. They also affect the brain; for example, blood flow fluctuations occur. These may be greater in the phase known as 'paradoxical sleep' than in wakefulness. Why paradoxical? Because the EEG looks more like that from an alert than from a sleeping person. There are also Rapid Eye Movements during this phase; hence the other name, REM sleep. If the subject is woken from this he will in most cases say that he has been dreaming and is able to recount dreams. This is rare in any other stage of sleep. Hence the idea that REM sleep is concerned with 'psychological restorative function'.

Sleep changes

The adult EEG is characterised by alpha activity over the posterior parts of the head. With the onset of drowsiness the alpha may in some individuals augment very briefly in amplitude before disappearing. The tracing is then characterised by widespread ragged low-amplitude activity of both fast and theta waves. Just as suddenly as it disappeared, the alpha may return. This transient appearance and disappearance of alpha can be likened to the waxing and waning of attention while listening to a boring lecture, or the brief moments in which the newspaper goes out of focus during a monotonous train journey to return to clear vision as the train suddenly rattles over points.

When the person has taken an oral hypnotic, this early stage of sleep may be very brief and within a few minutes of lying down on the EEG couch 'stage 2' sleep will supervene. It is characterised by a whole series of phenomena which are striking in their amplitude and shape (see Fig. 10.1), so much so that it is not surprising that in the early days of electroencephalography many were regarded as abnormal. There are three relatively localised phenomena, vertex sharp waves, so called because of their distribution around the vertex, sleep spindles or sigma rhythm, seen mainly over the frontal regions, and lambdoid waves, visible in the occipital areas. K complexes on the other hand are generalised. They consist of high-voltage delta waves appearing synchronously on the two sides preceded or followed by bursts of sleep

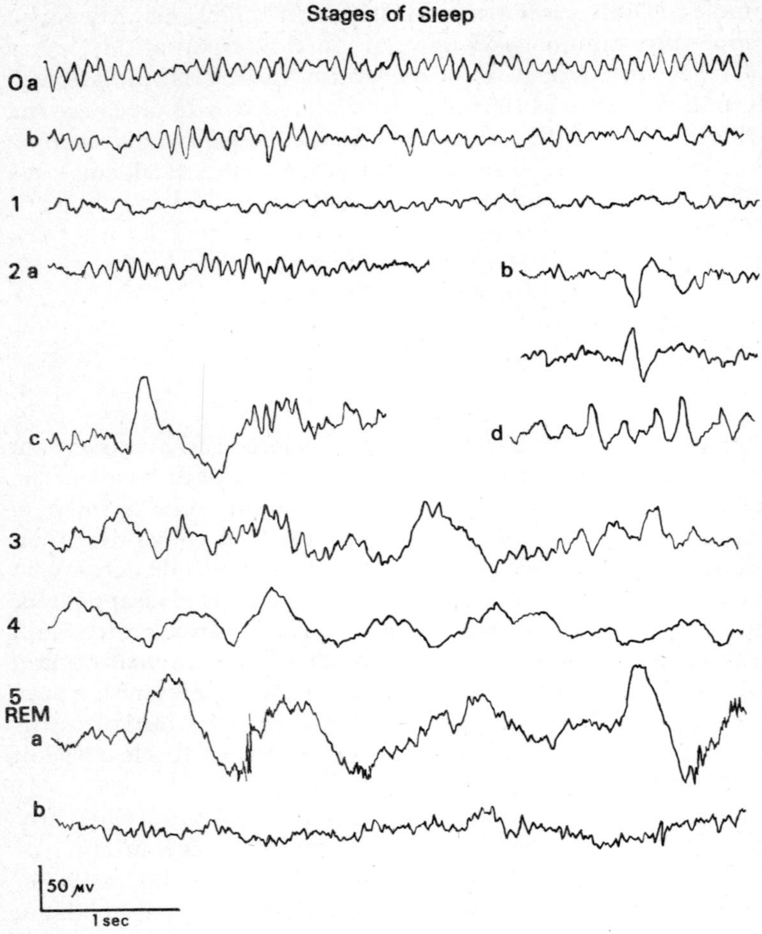

Figure 10.1 Sleep stages
0. (a) Continuous alpha activity (b) Alpha activity breaking up — drowsiness
1. Stage-1 sleep. Low amplitude record with fast components and some theta activity
2. Stage-2 sleep. (a) Sigma rhythm or spindles (b) Vertex sharp waves (c) K complex (d) Lambdoid waves
3. Stage-3 sleep. Delta activity with some sigma rhythm
4. Stage-4 sleep. Virtually continuous delta only
5. Stage REM. (a) Rapid eye movements monitored while (b) shows a low amplitude EEG not markedly dissimilar from 1

spindles. These complexes occur either spontaneously or in response to stimuli.

The deepest stages of sleep, labelled 3 and 4, occur about 45 minutes after sleep begins. These stages are defined in terms of the relative amounts of delta activity and stage-2 phenomena. These latter are completely absent in stage 4.

The next phase of sleep – the Rapid Eye Movement stage (REM) was not appreciated until relatively recently (Aserinsky and Kleitman 1955). The change from stage 4 is usually sudden. Widespread high-voltage irregular delta disappears, and the tracing is then of low voltage, showing little rhythmic activity. It is not dissimilar to the pattern seen in alert subjects, but there are two other features: clusters of rapid eye movements and an increase in muscle potentials. When long sleep recordings are carried out, in order to detect and quantify the amounts of the various sleep stages extra electrodes must be used. The vertical and horizontal eyeball movements are monitored by placing electrodes near the eyes, one a centimetre above the outer canthus of the left eye and another a centimetre below the outer canthus of the right eye. The potentials at these electrodes are referred to each mastoid process and written out as two channels on the EEG tracing. The muscle potentials are picked up with a pair of electrodes, stuck to the skin, one on either side of the neck below the jaw.

All night sleep record

Most of the recordings carried out in electrophysiological research on sleep last the whole night, the so called 'all night sleep record'. The sheer bulk of these EEGs, even when recorded at a slower paper speed than the 3 centimetres per second which is usual for routine work, still leads to tracings of daunting proportions.

As a result some laboratories have employed highly compressed and tape-recorded tracings using EEG channels, while the important physiological variables such as eye movement and muscle are combined in a single channel. Nevertheless, the ordinary ink-on-paper tracing is usual in most laboratories because it is convenient for visual assessment.

The tracings have to be rated page by page. This may be anything from ten seconds to two minutes of brain activity, depending on the paper speed. On the basis of the phenomena seen, the stage of sleep is determined and an approximate figure entered on a separate sheet for further analysis later, usually by computer.

In order to do the sleep staging accurately and with consistency, so that results from various centres can be compared, an atlas of tracings and detailed descriptions was drawn up by an international group (Rechtschaffen and Kales 1968). Another method of increasing accuracy is to have two or more people assessing the tracings independantly; later they compare their results, discussing and resolving any differences. Obviously, visual rating is a laborious process, and so methods of computer analysis are in various stages of development. It does appear, however, at the present time that the simple, if tedious 'eyeballing' technique is still the most accurate and widely used. Because of the cost of all-night sleep recording and the fact that the laboratory may almost entirely be taken up with this work, there are few centres. At the present time there is probably only one in the United Kingdom, run by Dr Ian Oswald in Edinburgh, though there are a large number in the United States and on the continent of Europe.

Psycho-physiological changes

Sleep is often divided into two sorts, the REM and the non-REM sleep, because there are a number of interesting psycho-physiological differences between the two types. The subject as he gets progressively deeper asleep passes through stages 1 to 4 and as he does so his respiration and heart-rate slow, the blood pressure falls, and there is a diminution in muscle tone. In addition, he is increasingly difficult to wake. REM sleep is characterised by irregularity and variability of the heart and respiration, and the blood pressure tends to rise, although muscle tone is markedly diminished; there are twitchings of face and limbs. The subject is difficult to rouse, but if awakened from this state he will recall dreams. During non-REM sleep subjects are rarely able to do this.

The pattern of the night's sleep is a cyclical one, periods of REM sleep recurring 4 to 5 times during the course of the 7 to 8 hours sleep in young adults. The first appearance of REM is usually an hour to an hour-and-a-half after sleep commences, and the total amount of the night's sleep spent in the REM stage is 20 to 25%, the REM stage recurring for periods of 20 minutes or so.

Just how important REM sleep is has not yet been finally established. It has been suggested that depletion of it leads to psychotic manifestations. This could be understood because the individual was deprived of dreaming, which occurs almost exclusively during REM sleep. However, the earlier claims about psychological disturbance have not been supported by subsequent research.

There is no doubt that most psychotropic drugs decrease the amount of REM sleep. Barbiturates have been studied in detail by Oswald and Priest (1965) and cause a decrease in the time taken to get to sleep, an increase in the amount of slow-wave sleep, but a decrease in the amount of REM. If the drug is continued, the amount of REM returns to its usual figure of 25% after a week or so – perhaps a neurophysiological parallel to the process of 'drug tolerance' familiar to pharmacologists. The stopping of the drug leads to a marked increase in the amount of REM sleep and it may take several weeks to return to normal. This 'REM rebound' was studied by Oswald and colleagues. They demonstrated that in normal subjects given a barbiturate for six nights and then withdrawn, even six nights later the amount of REM had still not returned to its normal base line.

Clinical use of all-night sleep recording

There are relatively few conditions in which an over-night sleep recording is required for clinical diagnosis. Narcolepsy is one example. This syndrome is characterised by cataplexy, sleep paralysis and hallucinosis, in addition to the cardinal symptom, an insatiable desire to sleep. The narcoleptic patient shows quite a different pattern at the onset of sleep from that seen in normals. He goes directly from waking into REM sleep (Parkes and Marsden 1974). Patients who suffer from hypersomnia, that is excessive sleeping without any of the additional features of narcolepsy, do not show this particular pattern. They follow the conventional route through stages 1 to 4 before they move into REM sleep. However, in these conditions it may be necessary to repeat the EEG on two or even three occasions in order to establish the diagnosis. Presumably the laboratory situation influences the patients' ability to sleep and they do not lapse into sleep until they are familiar with it.

In some patients with epilepsy overnight sleep recordings may help to establish the diagnosis, particularly if the patient is deprived of sleep on the night before the test is carried out. Epileptic discharges of a variety of different types may emerge when they have been absent in the routine scalp recording, in particular those arising in the amydala and hippocampal regions.

Other disorders in which disturbances of sleep patterns are found, but in whom the significance of the findings is as yet not established, include schizophrenia and noctural enuresis, while it is of interest that in alcohol withdrawal stages there is a great excess of REM sleep.

A new impetus has been given to the neurophysiological study of sleep by the realisation that striking changes occur in other bodily systems during REM sleep. There are rapid swings in blood pressure and this sometimes reaches much higher levels than observed in wakefulness, a change that, it is suggested, may cause nocturnal angina. Another type of change has been observed in the gastro-intestinal tract. Gastric mobility increases and probably the level of acid in the stomach. This may account for dyspeptic pain during sleep.

Sleep has also been studied in an attempt to determine the cause of delirium following surgery. It is a particular problem after heart operations which are often long and in which cardio-pulmonary by-pass has to be used. In these investigations sleep was monitored not just during the night but 'round the clock' before and after operation (Johns *et al.* 1974). The total sleep in these patients was reduced and very little REM sleep occurred at all, in contrast to the pattern in delirium from alcohol withdrawal or unconsciousness after suicidal attempts with central nervous depressant drugs (Gross *et al.* 1966, and Haider and Oswald 1970). These findings therefore suggest that there must be other factors in post-operative patients, not simply the effect, for example, of 'withdrawal from anaesthesia'.

The assessment of hypnotic drugs

Hypnotics are one of the most commonly prescribed compounds and it is generally recognised that there are marked individual variations in response to them. We have already seen how they may affect sleep profoundly, both during administration and after withdrawal. Because all-night sleep recordings are time-consuming and expensive, in the studies that I have carried out with colleagues on the assessment of hypnotics we have concentrated on records of 30 to 120 minutes duration. In addition to the EEG, we have used a number of other tests which give numerical data. For example, the subjective effects of a hypnotic were assessed using rating scales. Behavioural tests have been performed following administration of drugs, to determine whether they affected for example reaction time. In a number of investigations we have tested the blood levels of the drug during the actual EEG recording, using an in-dwelling needle, so that repeated blood samples could be obtained without disturbing the patient (Speirs *et al.* 1972).

The design of the studies themselves has always been careful. Usually two different drugs have been used, sometimes at different dose levels, and placebo has invariably been given in sequence. In addition, all the assessments including that of EEG have been carried out in a 'double blind' manner. The order in which the drugs and placebo were administered was balanced for the whole group so that any order effects or other extraneous variables were, as far as possible, cancelled out.

At the end of a study, when all the EEGs have been collected, they are masked, coded and rated, often by two raters independently. The particular method of EEG assessment is as follows: each page of the EEG, that is 10 seconds of the recording, is examined to determine what sleep stage the person was in during that period: if stage 1, the value '1' was assigned; if stage 3, the value '3' and so on. When the whole of the EEG had been rated the numbers could be dealt with in various ways. For example, a total score for the whole of the record would be equivalent to the depth and duration of sleep. Hence it was easy to determine whether one drug was more effective than another. The time taken to reach a particular depth of sleep could be obtained, and also how many changes from sleep to alertness occurred during a particular EEG. Using these methods it has been possible to show that even 18 hours after a single night-time dose of a hypnotic such as nitrazepam it still has effects on the EEG (Malpas *et al.* 1970). The subject was more likely to fall asleep during the recording than if he had taken a barbiturate such as amylobarbitone or placebo on the previous night. Interestingly enough behavioural testing showed that the patients were still 'slowed' some 12 hours following the administration of the hypnotic, although they were quite unaware of this. Using a similar technique we have shown that in anxious patients there is less tendency for this persistent effect (Malpas *et al.* 1974). We have also studied the hypnotic effects of anticonvulsant drugs in normal subjects and have shown that small doses of phenytoin are less sedative than phenobarbitone, which is quite understandable. More surprisingly, the subjects are more alert following phenytoin than placebo, confirming that phenytoin may have a mild CNS stimulant effect.

In these studies we have thus reduced complex EEG data into a simple numerical form, which can be assessed by the usual statistical means. Further we have shown that positive results can emerge when such EEG techniques are combined with a stringent methodological approach. Taken in a wider context, there is no doubt that EEG sleep studies are one of the major growing points of neurophysiology.

CHAPTER ELEVEN

Brain 'Death'

The brain of a living person produces electrical potentials, but that of a dead individual is electrically 'silent'. This type of EEG used to be called 'flat,' but the term has been employed widely to describe low-voltage arhythmic records which may be quite normal for an alert elderly subject. Hence the term 'isoelectric' is used nowadays.

An isoelectric EEG is regarded in some countries as essential for the diagnosis of death. This is unwise for two main reasons. First, the diagnosis of death should be made on the basis of clinical criteria, absent reflexes, no spontaneous respiration, failure to maintain blood pressure, and to this may be added in some circumstances the EEG information. Secondly, the isoelectric EEG may be seen in patients who subsequently recover full cerebral function, for example after suicidal barbiturate overdose. In addition the isoelectric EEG can come about from a great variety of causes – cardiac arrest, encephalitis, head injury, and hepatic encephalopathy to give a few examples.

There has nevertheless been an increasing interest recently in EEG, principally for two reasons: first, because of the development of transplant surgery, and in these circumstances the earlier the diagnosis of death is made the more likely is it that the organs will function satisfactorily in the recipient; secondly, because of the increasing interest in intensive care units. Obviously it is necessary to establish that patients undergoing this expensive (Skillman 1974) form of treatment will have adequate brain function if they recover. An important secondary issue here is the 'persistent vegetative state'. Methods by which the prognosis of severe cerebral insults could be predicted in order to avoid patients recovering only to this state of 'suspended animation' would be extremely valuable. Unfortunately at the present time it can be said that there is no means of accurate prediction about this either on clinical or on electroencephalographic grounds.

Technical considerations

It is often difficult to obtain satisfactory EEGs on patients in coma. The recordings must obviously be made at the bedside and not in the EEG department and generally there is other equipment near the patient, at least a respirator and often an array of monitoring devices, and these may make it difficult for the technician to get near enough even to the patient's head to apply the electrodes. In these circumstances we have favoured sterilised platinum needle electrodes which can be put quickly into place and yield a satisfactory recording. They also need little cleaning-up, in contrast to stick-on electrodes where collodion must be applied and then subsequently removed using acetone. Ideally two technicians are needed, and during part of the actual recording it is helpful and sometimes essential for the electroencephalographer to be present as well.

One of the problems could be regarded as 'philosophical'. We are as it were searching for 'nothing'. As a result we find a variety of artefacts which we have to distinguish from the 'real thing'. The sources of artefact (see Chapter 2) in this situation are similar to those seen in any EEG but are somewhat more troublesome. Mains hum from electrical apparatus by the patient's bedside may completely mask the tracing (see Fig. 11.1). Then movements of the patient's head with respiration or with each heart beat – the ballistocardiographic effect – may make the EEG particularly difficult to interpret.

The basic problem is that we wish to use the maximum amplification in order to display any low-voltage brain potentials, but the more we increase the amplification the more is the extraneous 'noise' amplified as well. This is a general problem of EEG. In ordinary recordings the signals from the brain are large and the background 'noise' is relatively small. The situation is quite different when there is little or no cerebral activity.

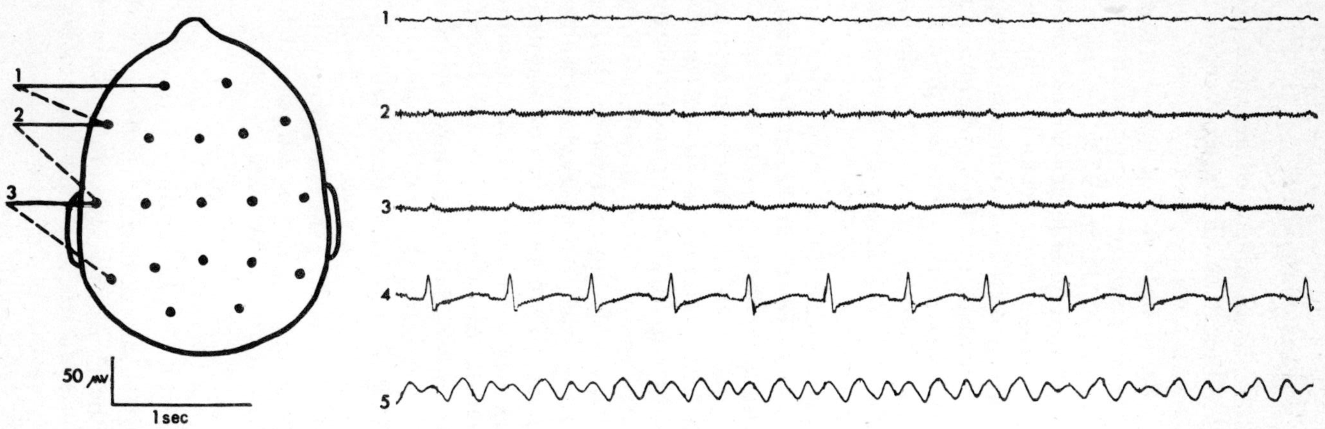

Figure 11.1 A totally isoelectric EEG 12 hours after a cardiac arrest. Note that channels 1, 2 and 3 have no cerebral activity but they show mains hum – 50 cycle, and cardiographic artefact. This can be checked by reference to channel 4 which is the classical lead 1 electrocardiograph. Channel 5 is the output from the transducer which is monitoring head movements

The difficulties of obtaining a technically satisfactory isoelectric EEG (see Fig. 11.1) have been recognised world-wide, and many countries have adopted their own particular standards. These need not concern us in detail as they have been discussed elsewhere (Pampiglione and Harden 1968, Silverman *et al.* 1969, Prior 1973). In essence, it is emphasised that there should be at least ten electrodes on the scalp, that the contact between the scalp and the electrodes should be satisfactory and that the recording apparatus should have at least four channels. The minimum of filtering should also be used and part of the recording should be taken with an increased sensitivity of at least 25 microvolts per centimetre. The effects of stimulation of the patient should be checked.

I personally insist that the cardiograph is run simultaneously with the EEG, at least for part of the recording. This is a simple check that the system is working satisfactorily. A biological signal arising from the patient emerging from the EEG machine indicates that there is continuity. In any case the cardiograph is often seen on the EEG leads when there are no cerebral potentials, and it is therefore necessary by eye to subtract the cardiograph from the cerebral channels in order to decide whether any cerebral activity is present or not. If there are other potentials which are probably artefactual then these can be monitored by placing a transducer on the appropriate part of the body. These small devices convert movement into electrical signals which are then written out on the tracing, so that the wave form can be compared directly with that recorded from the scalp electrodes. In this way it is possible to distinguish the real from the artefactual. If the respirator is causing disturbance on the tracing, this can be turned off for a brief period and respiration continued by hand.

The isoelectric EEG

Let us assume that we have obtained a satisfactory EEG and are certain that there are no cerebral potentials. What statement can be made to the clinician? We can say that the EEG is 'isoelectric', devoid of cerebral potentials, but what value can be placed on this particular statement? Under what circumstances could this type of tracing occur in a patient who will recover fully? The chances, taking all the 'ifs and buts' into consideration, are very small. In a series of cases reviewed by the American EEG Society only 3 out of 1665 patients recovered (Silverman *et al.* 1969). These were all patients who had taken overdoses of central nervous depressant drugs.

Table 11.1 The main items on the technicians' check list when recording at the bedside of a patient following a cardio-respiratory arrest

General:	Date and time of recording Ward Technician's name
Technical:	Type of machine and electrodes used Any fault noted in the apparatus
Artefacts:	Type seen and how monitored
Clinical:	Date and time of last arrest State of consciousness Respiration, spontaneous or assisted Vital functions, temperature, blood pressure etc. Seizures in preceding 24 hours, type and timing Metabolic state, recent electrolyte and urea values Drugs: nature, dosage and timing
Present state:	Level of arousal during recording Behavioural effects of stimulation Seizures observed Drugs given during the EEG

The actual check list used at the London Hospital is reproduced in Prior (1973).

If the circumstances of the 'collapse' are known – for example, a cardiac arrest – then much more weight can of course be placed on the EEG devoid of cerebral potentials. We have a check list (Prior 1973) (Table 11.1) filled in by the

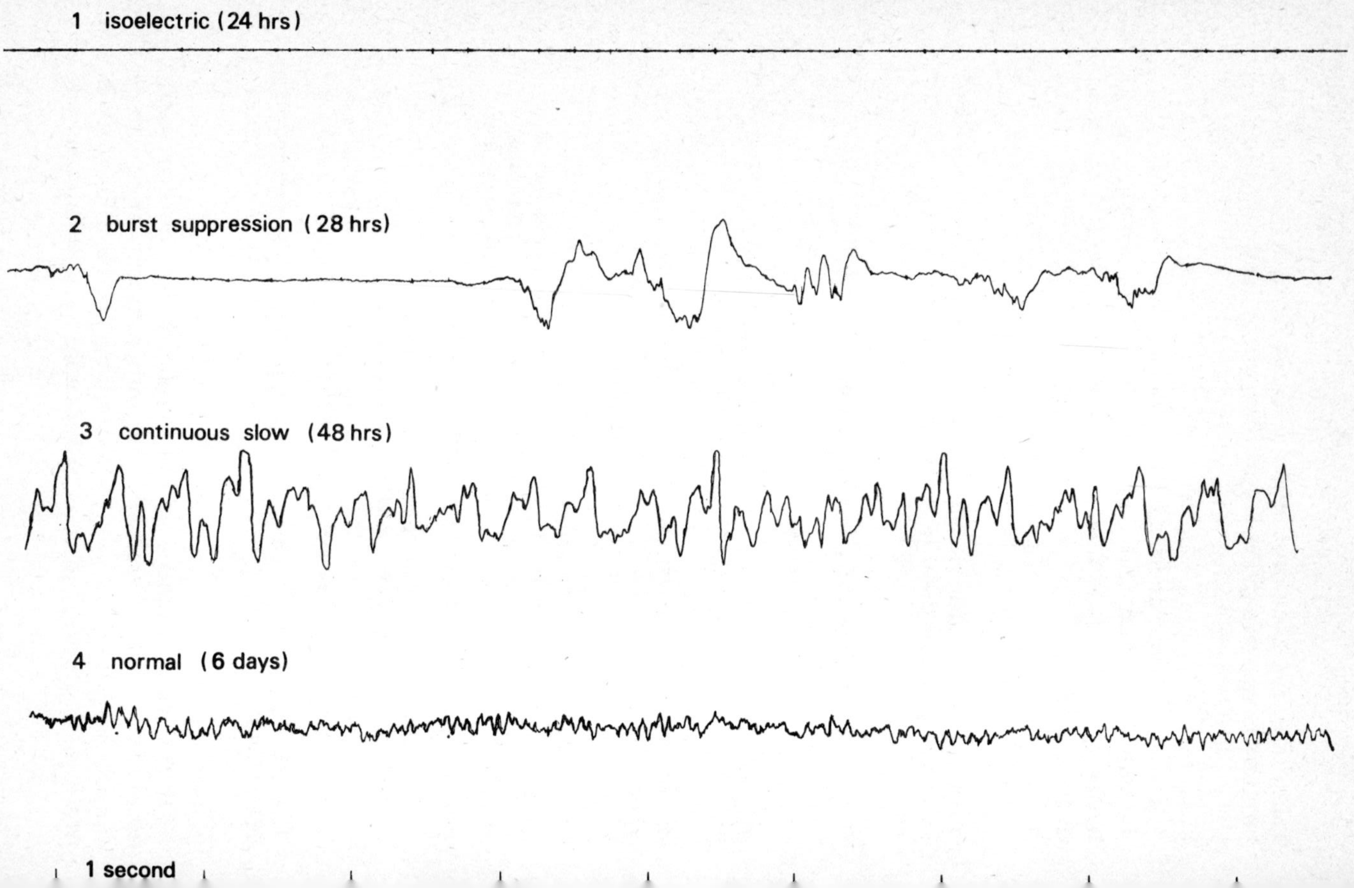
1 isoelectric (24 hrs)
2 burst suppression (28 hrs)
3 continuous slow (48 hrs)
4 normal (6 days)
1 second

Figure 11.2 The EEG during recovery from barbiturate overdose. The recording is totally isoelectric 24 hours after the overdose. Four hours later discontinuous activity is re-appearing and then section 3 at 48 hours shows continuous activity. Six days following the overdose the EEG has returned to normal

technician at the time of taking the EEG so that we are aware of the patient's blood pressure, temperature, metabolic state and so on where the EEG is reported.

In general, care with the prognostic statement on an isoelectric EEG must be taken when the patient has had a recent head injury, or had recent major fits, or is known to have severe electrolyte or metabolic disorder. Also, if the patient is hypothermic one also has reservations, although even with temperatures of below 20° Centigrade the recording may not be totally isoelectric if the brain has not been damaged in any way previously.

Because of these various 'ifs and buts' it is usual to say that the EEG should be repeated in 12 to 24 hours and this is a fairly generally accepted standard. The American EEG Society suggest two recordings of 30 minutes duration 24 hours apart. As we shall see later, it may be possible to give a more definite prognostic statement on the basis of a single EEG.

Drug coma

The one exception to the serious prognostic importance of an isoelectric EEG is in drug induced coma (see Fig. 11.2). After, for example, a suicidal overdose with barbiturates or other CNS depressant drugs, the EEG may be absolutely devoid of cerebral potentials and remain so for as long as 30 hours; yet the patient may recover fully. It is therefore essential in patients in whom the history is unclear to determine blood levels of barbiturates and other drugs before resuscitative measures are withdrawn. However, the situation is more complicated even in patients with barbiturate coma, for they may show cerebral activity, and in any case they may have suffered periods of severe hypotension or even cardiac arrest. Therefore, even in the presence of central nervous depressant drugs, circulating in the blood and

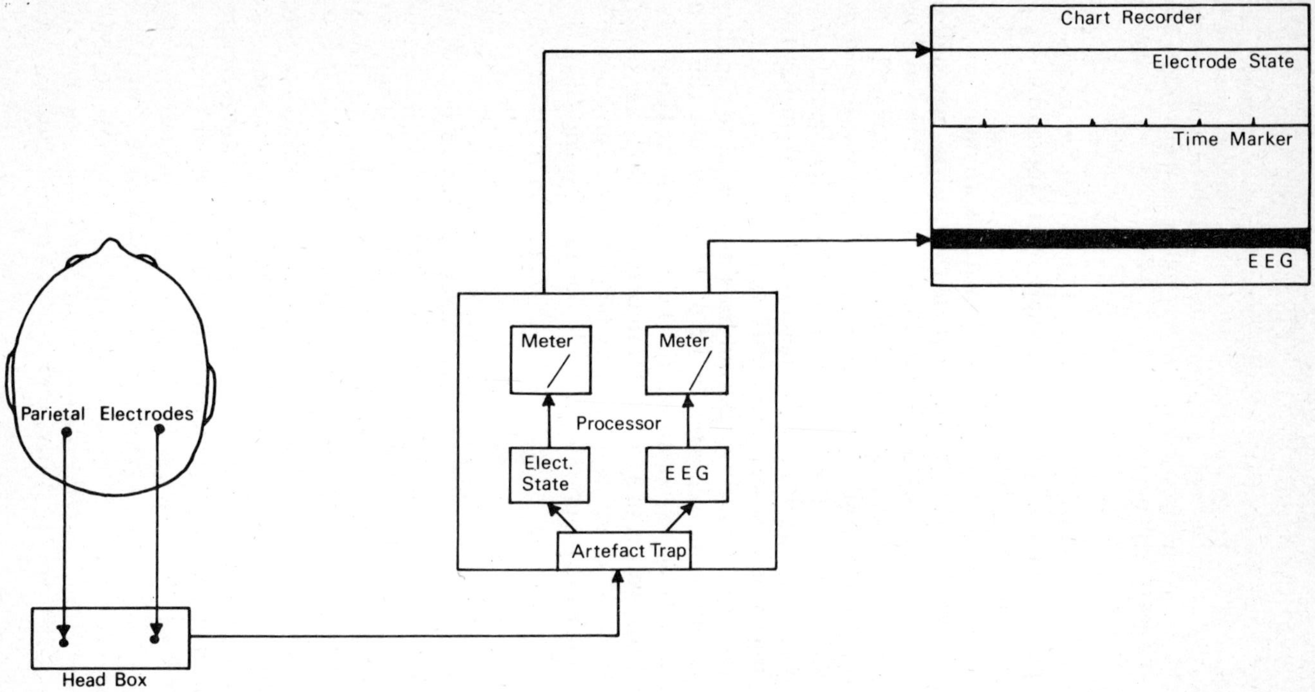

Figure 11.3 Block diagram of the Cerebral Function Monitor (CFM)

reaching the brain, the outlook must often be guarded in the early stages.

The Cerebral Function Monitor (CFM)

Let us for the moment consider what the EEG is. As it lasts only 20 to 30 minutes it is merely a 'snap shot' of brain activity. It is conceivable that the EEG may be isoelectric in the morning and that activity may return in the afternoon. Ideally, we need a way of monitoring cerebral activity continuously rather than taking a 'snap shot' every 24 hours. For this reason a simple monitoring device was invented at the London Hospital by Maynard (Maynard *et al.* 1969, Prior *et al.* 1971). It uses a single pair of electrodes and produces a compressed EEG recording which can be kept running for hours or even days. The paper trace is much shorter than the conventional EEG; the former is produced at the rate of 10 cms per hour, the latter usually at 3 cms per sec. Although it has been used in patients with cardiac arrest, there are a number of other situations in which it may be valuable: for example, during open heart surgery when cerebral perfusion may be vulnerable to impairment.

The device (see Fig. 11.3) consists of two parallel systems, one for processing the EEG signal and the other for indicating the state of the recording electrodes. There is a single pair of ordinary stick-on electrodes attached by a screened cable to the CFM. The EEG signal is filtered, so that unwanted potentials are rejected, and it is then amplified and compressed. The write-out is in the form of a dark band produced by a hot-wire recorder. The lower limit of the band represents the lowest level of cerebral activity in terms of microvolts and the width of the band indicates the variability of the cerebral activity. Certain patterns emerge which we learn to recognise by comparing them with the full conventional EEG. Subsequently, it has been possible to say what the cerebral activity is like directly from inspection of the CFM tracing. The state of the electrodes in the form of 'impedance' is written out on a second parallel trace so that poor contact or other problems are shown by a change in the tracing.

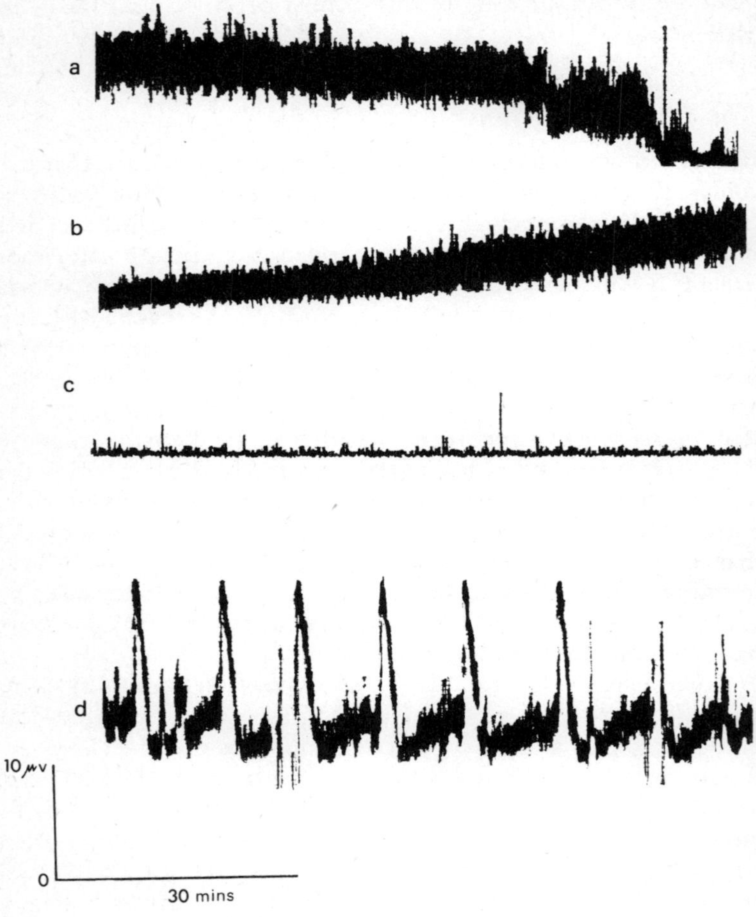

Figure 11.4 Examples of Cerebral Function Monitor tracings
(a) Decline in cerebral activity and finally death following cardiac arrest
(b) Gradual increase in cerebral activity as may be seen in a patient recovering from a barbiturate overdose
(c) A persistently near-zero level tracing, in a patient whose conventional EEG is isoelectric
(d) A series of stereotyped 'sharp waves' associated with clinical seizures

Various types of trace have been seen, and they fall into three main groups (see Fig. 11.4). The first, the sustained near-zero level, is important in patients following cardiac arrest. The trace is rarely absolutely on the baseline due to slight pick-up of muscle potentials and other artefacts which can enter even though the instrument has a high rejection factor. If the tracing remains at a near-zero level for 24 hours between two conventional isoelectric EEG recordings, one can be certain that there has been no abrupt change in cerebral activity. A second type of pattern is one in which there is either a marked up-swing or down-swing. The former occurs, for example, during recovery from barbiturate coma, a change which may precede clinical improvement, and the latter in, for example, a patient with a failing heart and decreasing cerebral perfusion.

The third group of changes, in contra-distinction to the second group, are sudden, occurring over a period of minutes rather than hours. If a CFM recording is in progress and an episode of cardiac arrest occurs with quick resuscitation, then a sudden fall to base line with recovery to the pre-existing level is seen. Seizures also show sudden changes, and a variety of different patterns can, with experience be discerned.

EEG assessment of outcome after cardiac arrest

The CFM obviously adds new information on the EEG in unconscious patients, but the main problem still remains, how to relate particular EEG features to a favourable or unfavourable outcome, as well as to determine just how early it is possible to give a prediction as to the ultimate prognosis. To this end a series of more than 300 unconscious patients after resuscitation have been studied at the London Hospital. A hundred of these showed no cerebral activity at any stage (Prior *et al.* 1974). None of the patients in whom there was persistent isoelectric EEGs survived for more than 2 or 3 weeks, although instances of 5 months' survival do occur (Brierley *et al.* 1971). None of these patients is living in the ordinary sense of the word. They show merely reflex responses. Of the 35 patients of Prior and colleagues who had isoelectric recordings in the first 24 hours, 32 died without regaining consciousness; only 3 survived, one with severe residual brain damage, while two recovered fully. One of these patients was in coma following a barbiturate overdose. Let us now consider patients who do have cerebral activity. The EEG following, for example, a cardiac arrest may show a wide range of different types of phenomena. There may be present slow-wave activity, repetitive complexes, sharp waves, or a burst-suppression pattern – that is, clusters of activity separated by periods when no potentials can be seen, like those in Fig. 11.2, sections 2 and 3. Because of the profusion of different types of abnormality and the fact that they may be seen differently over the two hemispheres, assessment by visual inspection is made complex. In addition, prognostication is difficult.

It was for this reason that, almost ten years ago, we began developing in conjunction with colleagues elsewhere a system whereby the EEG phenomena seen in these records could not only be noted but also rated in terms of their amount. In all, about 50 EEG features were assessed and two raters worked independently. In addition, two clinical items were added, namely the time after the cardiac arrest that the EEG had been taken and the patient's clinical responsiveness during the EEG. The outcome in 41 patients, from whom 93 EEGs were recorded, was determined in detail – whether they died or survived, and whether the death was a cerebral one. Moreover in some instances neuro-pathological information was available to confirm the presence or absence of cerebral anoxia. These data were subjected to a discriminant function analysis. With so many variables, a computer was used. The aim of the computer analysis was to pick out those factors which are likely to have predictive value about outcome. The advantage of this type of analysis is that it gives an indication of the relative importance of various changes. It showed us, somewhat unexpectedly, that phenomena which occurred repeatedly throughout the EEG, particularly those with a regular periodicity, carried a bad prognosis. Rather surprisingly the dominant frequency of the EEG activity did not figure largely in predicting outcome. On general grounds one would have thought an EEG with delta activity was worse than one in which there was theta activity, and similarly this would be a worse sign than if alpha was dominant. In fact, the amplitude of activity was a more important parameter, with consistently low amplitude of 10 to 20 microvolts being a particularly unfavourable sign. This study (Binnie *et al.* 1970) showed that complex EEG data can be conveniently analysed using a computer, and it was possible to make accurate predictions about outcome on a single EEG in over 95% of instances. If serial EEGs are taken into consideration the prediction can be even more accurate. The problem remains, however, that it is not possible to use this technique without recourse to a computer. Hence the next development.

A similar set of data was analysed in a different way using an adaptive discriminant function analysis (Maynard and Prior 1973). In essence a computer program is used which not only tests which variables predict outcome in terms of death or survival but successively discards those which do not help to discriminate. Thus our original 50 variables were reduced to 13. Of these there were two clinical features, response to stimulation and time since the cardiac arrest, and the remainder were EEG features which have to be rated according to clearly defined criteria in terms of the phenomena present and the amount. Following these calculations on the computer it was possible to build a desk-top device (the survival predictor) with a series of 13 complex switches, each of which had several positions indicated by numbers on the switches. These are set in turn as the EEG is assessed visually. For example, if alpha is absent the switch concerned with the alpha rating is set at '0'. If there is a moderate amount of alpha activity the setting is '4'. The same applies to the other features. This device allows us immediately after the EEG has been rated to compare it with previous experience on the outcome of patients with cerebral anoxia following cardiac arrest, as there is a meter on the device which indicates whether the score is characteristic of recovery or 'brain death'. Further, the apparatus indicates whether the EEG under consideration is typical of others previously examined. Sometimes the patients who are 'atypical' turn out to have other confusing clinical factors which have not been appreciated at the time the EEG was taken.

The added advantage of this device is that, should there be any doubt about the presence of a particular EEG feature or its amount, the effect on the meter of various settings of the switch in question can be tested. The device can therefore add to our confidence when giving the EEG report which in no way replaces this. Using all these techniques together, it appears that a prognostic statement about outcome can be made as early as six hours after a cerebral anoxic episode (Prior *et al.* 1974), but more data are needed before an absolutely definitive statement is possible.

To conclude, it can be seen that some of the problems relating to the EEG and cerebral death have been solved, in spite of the complexity of the data. This has been possible with the use of specialised techniques for quantifying the EEG phenomena, of continuous monitoring and of the 'survival predictor'. These have all added to the accuracy of assessments. This is not to say that further progress cannot be made. The particular problem relates to quality of survival in those patients who have suffered cerebral anoxia. Will they have severe and persistent cerebral damage and therefore end in a 'persistent vegetative state', or will they recover with only minor degrees of abnormality compatible with relatively normal life? Further studies are obviously required in many centres and these are continuing in our laboratory as well.

CHAPTER TWELVE

Anaesthetics and the EEG

There has been a close interaction between anaesthesia and electroencephalography since the earliest days of the technique. Indeed Berger, the discoverer of EEG, reported in 1933, four years after his original description of the human EEG, that chloroform changed the pattern (see Gloor 1969). Investigators in that early period included the Gibbs's and their associates. They described alterations during anaesthesia and suggested that it might be possible to correlate the biochemical effects of this with the recorded cerebral potentials. Since that time there has been a continuing relationship between electroencephalography and anaesthesia, sometimes with a love-hate quality. Nevertheless electroencephalography has figured as an important tool in anaesthetics both in research and clinical practice.

Recently, with the discovery of a number of new anaesthetic agents, including ketamine and alphaxalone-alphadolone (Althesin), there has been a considerable resurgence in investigation involving EEG both in animals and in humans. Further studies have continued on EEG as a means of assessing the state of cerebral integrity during major surgical procedures, especially those involving cardio-pulmonary by-pass.

What exactly does the electroencephalographer have to offer the anaesthetist? (Table 12.1). The answer is: in particular the assessment of anaesthetic agents, as well as the monitoring of cerebral potentials during surgery, and also in the Intensive Care Unit following such conditions as head injury, cardiac arrest and barbiturate over-dosage.

Effects of anaesthetic agents

From the practical point of view we can consider all

Table 12.1 EEG and the anaesthetist

1. Pre- and post-operative assessment of patients' cerebral state
2. Monitoring during surgery to assess (a) level of anaesthesia (b) cerebral perfusion during cardiac-pulmonary by-pass, hypothermia, and hypotension
3. Assessment of anaesthetic compounds, e.g. testing of new induction agent
4. Intensive therapy unit monitoring, e.g. following cardiac arrest, barbiturate overdose, and head injury
5. Assessment of prolonged light anaesthesia, e.g. in semi-conscious patients requiring ventilation following chest injury

anaesthetic agents together. As soon as induction of anaesthesia is commenced, individual differences in the EEG disappear, as well as regional differentiation of activity. Thus in the alert adult alpha occurs at the back of the head, whereas in a moderate level of anaesthesia delta is widespread and equal at the front and the back. This 'ironing out' of the EEG means of course that it is possible to obtain useful information with a limited electrode placement even with a single pair of electrodes, a point to which we shall return later. The changes provoked by anaesthesia include, early on, the augmentation of the voltage of activity with a decrease in frequency (see Fig. 12.1). Thus with the induction alpha activity disappears, to be followed successively by theta and delta components. Then there follows another change: activity becomes discontinuous, with generalised bursts of cerebral potentials followed by stretches of EEG lasting one or many seconds in which virtually no activity is seen, the burst-suppression pattern. Finally, in the very deepest stages of anaesthesia there is virtually no activity at all, the isoelectric EEG. The maintenance of consciousness depends on interaction between the cerebral cortex and the reticular formation. It follows therefore that anaesthetic agents have an action in both of these sites to varying degrees. This may account for the differences between the EEG pattern and the apparent clinical depths of anaesthesia with different types of agent. It has been suggested that anaesthetics owe their action to synaptic block in the reticular formation (Magoun 1963), but certain agents such as ketamine and thiopentone, when given, induce fast activity over the

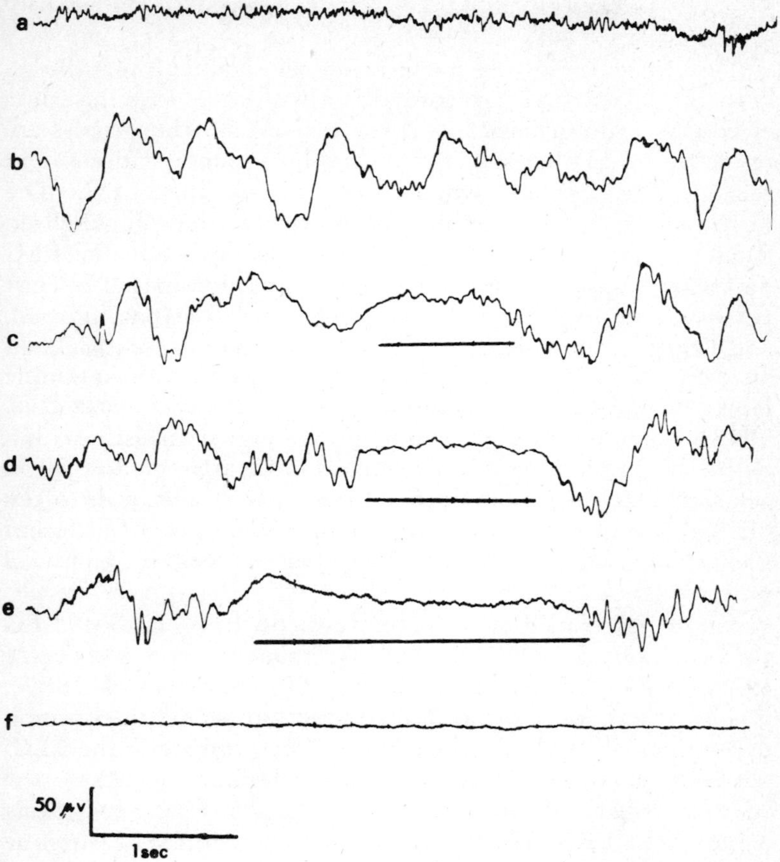

Figure 12.1 Changes following administration of an intravenous anaesthetic agent – thiopentone
(a) A 'desynchronised' EEG from a patient tense before induction of an anaesthetic
(b) High-voltage delta activity with superimposed fast elements occurring about one minute following injection
(c) The first sign of the EEG becoming 'discontinuous' as shown by underlining about 1½ minutes following injection
(d) An increased duration of suppression with almost total 'flattening' (underlined) in this instance about 2½ minutes following injection
(e) Almost total flattening (underlined) lasting nearly two seconds
(f) Total flattening lasting up to 10 seconds, the stage of deep surgical anaesthesia 4 or 5 minutes following the injection

cerebral cortex, an effect usually considered to be directly on the cortex itself.

The difficulty of comparing clinical depth of anaesthesia with the type of EEG recorded is a real one. Nowadays it is even more problematical, since a variety of other agents are used by anaesthetists, for example pre-medications and relaxants, some of which may affect the EEG. The introduction of ketamine in particular has highlighted discrepancies between the level of anaesthesia and the EEG pattern because this leads to a recording dominated by fast activity and theta components. This is somewhat unusual, and Coursen and colleagues (1969) used the term 'dissociated anaesthesia' because of this. However, even with ketamine larger doses cause a burst-suppression pattern (Schwartz *et al.* 1974), corresponding to a moderate depth of anaesthesia if a barbiturate anaesthesia had been given. Clearly the dose of an agent has to be taken into consideration, and it is often difficult to determine what are comparable doses of different compounds, especially when first introduced into clinical practice.

There is considerable literature on the various EEG patterns obtained with various anaesthetic agents (for example Faulconer and Bickford 1960, Sadove *et al.* 1967). As, however, most intravenous induction agents in common use are not dissimilar in the pattern they produce in the EEG, we have employed quantification techniques to assess the speed of onset of anaesthesia and the depth of anaesthesia achieved in EEG terms. This technique is similar to the one described for hypnotic agents (see Chapter 10). First of all, we define operationally the various EEG stages of anaesthesia and label them on a numerical scale. Then we go through the EEG recording studying each page – 10 seconds of EEG – quite separately, giving a numerical value depending on the activity seen. These numbers are added together to give a figure which corresponds to both depth and duration of anaesthesia. The speed of onset of anaesthesia can be defined as the time taken to reach a certain pre-specified level. In one study (Scott and Virden 1972) we found that there were small differences in the speed of onset of thiopentone anaesthesia compared with Althesin and we obtained values for the level reached. This study also showed the difficulty of judging equipotent doses of anaesthetic agents.

In another study (Schwartz *et al.* 1974) we compared the rate of onset of anaesthesia following ketamine injection, both with a conventional EEG and using a single channel device – the Cerebral Function Monitor (CFM) (see Chapter 11) and found the beginning of the drug effect was easier to determine on the CFM tracing than the conventional EEG.

The EEG has also been used to control the dose of anaesthetic. The technique is simple. The EEG is monitored and the signal obtained is passed into the anaesthetic machine. The dose of agent administered to the patient is adjusted automatically as the EEG changes. Thus, if the patient shows the pattern equivalent to deep anaesthesia, the dose of the compound is reduced, and vice versa. This ingenious method proposed by Faulconer and Bickford (1960), has not been widely adopted but could have a place, for example, in animal experiments, where a steady level of anaesthetic may be required over a long period of time while complex surgical procedures are undertaken.

Pre- and post-operative assessment

The EEG may be helpful in the pre-operative assessment of patients where there is a suspicion of cerebral pathology. Especially we have found this to be so in patients undergoing cardio-pulmonary by-pass. The pre-operative EEG forms a base-line against which post-operative tracings can be compared. For example, if it was known that there was an abnormality in the left temporal region related to a previous embolic episode, then EEG asymmetry in the post-operative period would not necessarily be interpreted as indicating that some untoward event had happened during surgery. The pre-operative EEG can also be of value when months after the operation the patient develops some cerebral symptoms or mental disorder. If another recording is performed and it differs markedly from the pre-operative tracing, then it is clear that either some new pathology has arisen or some damage has occurred during operation or in the post-operative period, perhaps not recognised at the time.

Monitoring during the operation

The EEG can be used to monitor cerebral activity during a variety of different types of operative procedure, for example those involving hypotension or hypothermia and in some instances during neurosurgical or cardiovascular procedures. We have been particularly interested in monitoring during open heart surgery; recently, using the CFM (see Chapter 10). This produces a compressed tracing from a single pair of electrodes. It has the advantage that the record can be easily interpreted 'on line' and the apparatus itself is less bulky than the conventional recording devices and does not need continuous skilled attention. We endeavoured to assess from the operative tracing the outcome in a hundred patients (Schwartz *et al.* 1973). Tracings were examined independently of their clinical outcome and placed into various categories, those with full clinical recovery, those with mild or moderate neurological sequelae and those with severe and irreversible cerebral damage. Eighty-five per cent of the tracings were categorised correctly. Such a blind assessment is of value in many contexts of EEG work, since it reduces the subjective element in the assessment and also allows us to establish more exact criteria. The CFM tracing is especially useful in this respect since changes can be measured simply with a ruler, a method which is quite impossible with the complex multi-channel recordings.

We have already given in detail the use of EEG monitoring in patients with cerebral hypoxia, but there are other conditions in which it may also be of value, either the single channel CFM or intermittent EEG recordings of conventional type: in patients with, for example, head injury, or in those with major injuries affecting the chest in which cerebral hypoxia or hypotensive complications may arise. One special case is the use of light continuous anaesthesia in order to maintain a patient with a serious chest injury in a state in which he will tolerate artificial ventilation. Here Ramsay and colleagues (1974) have reported the use of an Althesin drip and in these circumstances continuous assessment of the level of anaesthetic using the CFM is under study.

In this chapter some of the uses of EEG that can be made by anaesthetists have been given. The examples are by no means exhaustive and there are many problems in which the EEG could be usefully employed. One example has already been given in Chapter 10 where the amount and type of sleep following surgery has been assessed (Johns *et al.* 1974). If particular problems are clearly defined and the methodology of the study properly designed, so that subjective factors both on the clinical and EEG side can be reduced, there is no doubt that electroencephalography has a great deal to offer anaesthetists.

CHAPTER THIRTEEN

The Use of Evoked Response Techniques

Cerebral activity is minute in absolute terms, and this is even more noticeable because other deflections seen in the EEG, arising for example from eye movements, are very much larger. Thus the electroencephalographer by experience comes to ignore these artefactual phenomena, which can be regarded as 'noise', and evaluates only the potentials arising from the brain – the 'signals'. Most routine EEG work involves the consideration of on-going spontaneous cerebral activity. However, there is quite a different approach: namely, the evaluation of the effects of stimuli arriving in the brain and the observation of the cerebral potentials that result – the evoked responses. Generally, these responses are small and quite invisible by 'eye-balling', because they are intermingled with the on-going cerebral activity. Here the evoked response is the 'signal' and it bears a constant time relationship to the stimulus. The background on-going EEG is the 'noise'.

'Signal' and 'noise'

The problem of picking out small signals from the background of noise is not special for EEG. It is familiar to the radar engineer and the seismologist. Both send out signals and look at the returning 'echoes'. As with cerebral evoked responses, so with these echoes they bear a *constant* time relationship to the stimulus, and it is this fact which is the clue to a means of displaying them clearly. That is picking out the 'signal' from the background 'noise'. A simple way of doing this was proposed by Dawson (1947). The technique employed was that of photographic superimposition. The portion of the recording following the stimulus was displayed on a cathode ray oscilloscope and photographed. The next stimulus triggered the sweep of the cathode ray oscilloscope and once again the EEG was displayed and photographed on the same plate and so on for a run of stimuli. In this way the recurring wave form of the evoked response following the stimulus emerged from the blur of the constantly varying background activity which bore no definite time relationship to the stimulus. This superimposition technique can only be used when the responses are larger than or about the same size as the background noise.

The superimposition technique is relatively cumbersome, and subsequent methods have mostly relied upon computers, either small pre-programmed computers known as 'averagers' because they store the responses and average them at the end of each series of stimuli, or digital computers specially programmed for the purpose. Using these computer techniques even signals as small as one hundredth of the on-going noise can be detected. Nevertheless, the principle is similar to the superimposition method. The computer adds up consecutive samples of EEG trace following stimuli and, just like the cathode ray oscilloscope sweep, the computer is triggered by the stimulus. Once again the stimulus point is used for 'lining up' the traces, and after one EEG sample is collected and stored the computer gets ready to receive the next sample. As the series of stimuli continues the response becomes more obvious because it is time-locked to the stimulus, whereas the on-going EEG activity which has no constant relationship with the stimulus gradually cancels itself out (Fig. 13.1). In the end the response is quite obvious, appearing on a relatively 'noiseless' background. The result of each series of stimuli is displayed in a graphical form by a plotter. A block diagram of the apparatus is shown in Fig. 13.2 and for a more detailed technical exposition Cooper *et al.* (1974) should be consulted.

The method has a great advantage over the ordinary EEG with its wealth of data, some of which are redundant. The responses are relatively simple. Thus the technique represents a method of 'data reduction' which is extremely useful because the resulting plots are easy to analyse, and the deflections can be measured simply by a ruler. The response, for example, to different types of patterned visual material

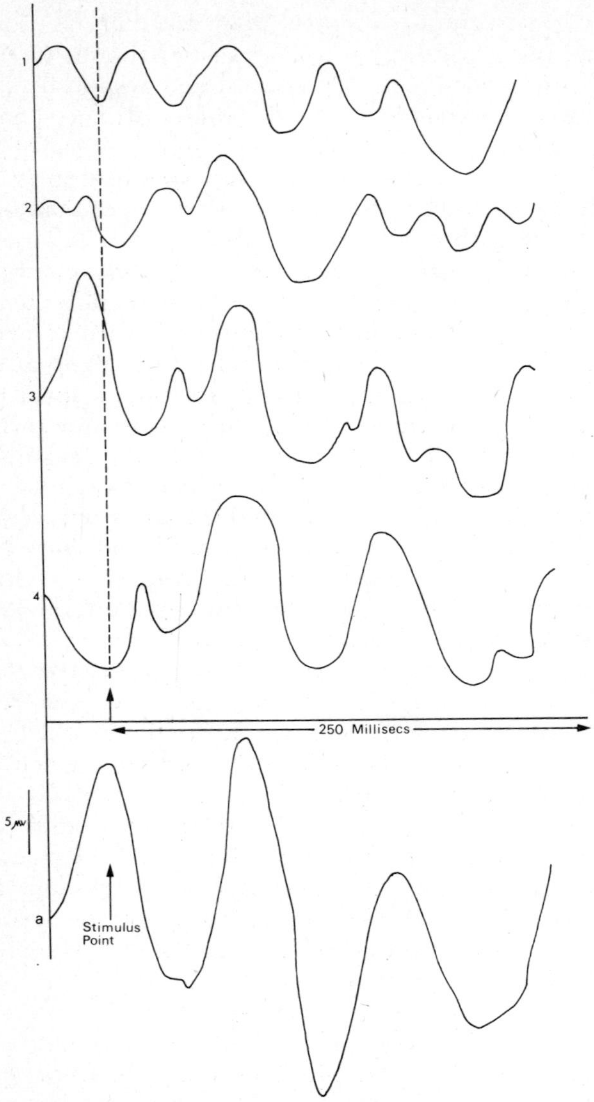

Figure 13.1 A demonstration of the principle of averaging. Each of the runs of activity labelled 1 to 4 is the small response to a single flash of light (retraced from originals). Looking at each individually there is no very clear cut response. However, when a further series of responses to a total of 32 flashes is 'averaged' a response like that at a. may be obtained. If one now runs one's eye back over the runs of activity labelled 1 to 4 the response 'buried in' the on-going activity can readily be discerned. This is the principle of averaging

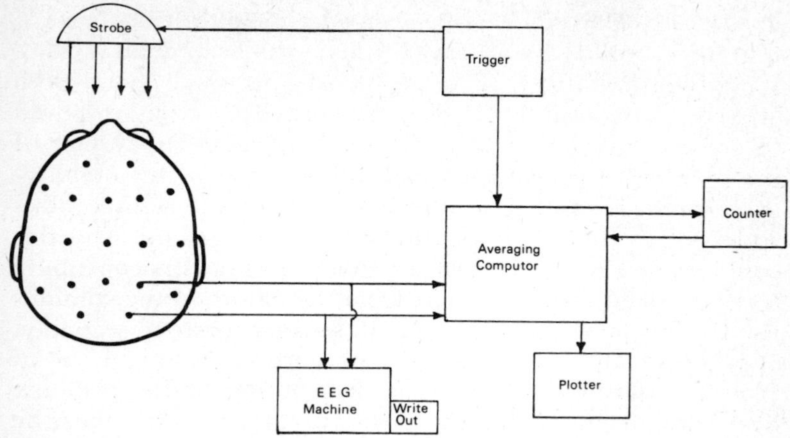

Figure 13.2 Block diagram of the apparatus for carrying out visual-evoked responses. Other types of response require only slight modification of the apparatus. Note that during 'averaging' the on-going cerebral activity is monitored with an EEG machine. In this way it is possible to make sure that there is no marked movement or other type of artefact which even though it tends to be diminished by averaging may not be entirely eliminated and may contaminate the evoked response

(Scott and Bickford 1969), different intensities of light, or the effect of monocular stimulation (Scott *et al.* 1969) can be compared simply by observation or by measurement. Thus we can determine the amplitude of particular components and the time at which they occur following the stimulus – the latency. Averaging techniques, however, have a disadvantage in that slight changes in wave form which may occur between the responses of a particular series are lost. More advanced methods, on the other hand, reveal that there are many components with various physiological significance, and they give not only the average wave form but also a measure of variability of the response over the series of stimuli.

Averages

The use of 'commercial' averages has had a great impact on electroencephalography. Since they became readily available in the early 1960s they have been employed to study cortical responses evoked by various stimuli of visual, auditory and somatosensory type. Even responses to smell have been assessed. The results of all this work have been reviewed recently in a comprehensive fashion by Regan (1972). One of the problems that emerged early on was the great variability of responses, so that results reported from various centres appeared to be conflicting. In order to understand why this could come about we must consider what factors contribute to the evoked response apart from the nature of the stimulus itself: first, the specific area of sensory cortex; secondly, changes in the adjacent areas of cortex; thirdly, level of arousal. Another factor is the distribution of the response over the cortex. Hence the positions of electrodes must be carefully studied, especially since Lehtinen and Bergstrom (1970) have shown that visual responses can be recorded even from the orbital surface of the frontal lobe. Because of variability it is not only useful but essential that a particular department should establish norms for its type of stimuli, electrode placements and apparatus. If we consider visual stimulation, the stroboscope used in one set of studies might be quite different from another in terms of whether the flash of light has a patterned quality or not. This relatively subtle variation in the stimulus leads to marked response differences which were not at first appreciated; nor were individual variations or alterations referable to changes of level of arousal of the subjects. Another factor is the age of the subject which of course applies to ordinary on-going EEG as well.

Clinical applications

It is probably because of this variability that clinical applications of these techniques have been relatively late, and at the present time there is much to be done in terms of the evaluation of the methods and their clinical usefulness. In this context the evoked response can be thought of simply as a means of testing the 'wiring' of a particular system in the CNS without the individual having to make a behavioural response.

An example is the investigation of an hysterically blind patient. If we find that there are normal visual-evoked responses over both occipital regions, then we have strong support for the view that the disturbance from which the patient complains is 'functional' rather than 'organic', as the pathways from the eyes to the visual cortex do not seem to be impaired. It is not possible of course to say that the patient can see, but at least the 'wiring' is in order. A similar approach applies to the testing of, for example, a possibly deaf brain-damaged child who cannot co-operate with the usual type of audiometry. We can test that the auditory evoked responses are present by what has come to be called 'cortical audiometry' (Cody *et al.* 1967) to see whether the responses are similar on the two sides and have a normal configuration. It is also possible to find at what intensity of sound they appear, that is we can obtain a hearing threshold (Taylor 1974). Recent studies have shown that it is even possible to record responses directly from the cochlear nerve itself (Solomon and Elberling 1971).

One particular clinical application for the visual-evoked response of great interest to neurologists is the testing of patients with retro-bulbar neuritis (Halliday *et al.* 1972). Here a patterned visual stimulus is used. It consists of an alternating chequer board, the black squares of which are replaced by white, and vice versa, twice a second. This can be done either mechanically by physically moving the board by the size of a square twice a second, or by other means, for example, the use of two slide projectors, each with two similar chequer boards but with the reverse pattern. The projectors are turned off and on at the rate of twice a second giving the same effect as the mechanical movement. The patient meanwhile fixates on a small spot at the centre of the pattern.

Patients with active optic neuritis show evoked responses which are diminished in amplitude or even absent, and the latency of a particular wave following the stimulus is markedly delayed by at least 20 milliseconds. The amplitude increases gradually as the neuritis subsides. However, the delayed latency persists indefinitely even though the basic condition improves (Fig. 13.3). This can be of great

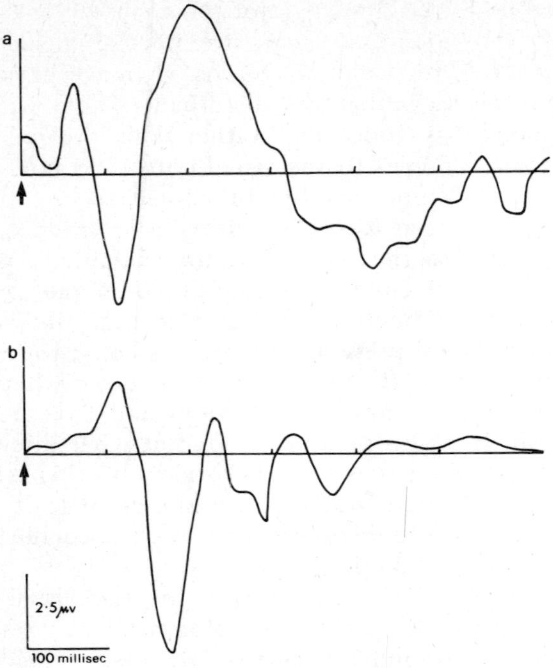

Figure 13.3 Visual evoked responses over the left occipital region to trains of 64 flashes with both eyes open. The arrows indicate moment of stimulation (responses retraced from originals)
(a) A normal subject. Note downgoing positive deflection at 100 milliseconds
(b) Patient with a history of retrobulbar neuritis. Note that the main deflection is displaced to the right compared with (a); that is, delayed to about 180 milliseconds after the flash

diagnostic significance, when a patient later develops a paraparesis of unknown aetiology. The visual-evoked responses are tested, and if there is a delay it is indicative of a previous episode of demyelination and would support the view that the present condition is a further episode of demyelination. These techniques in patients with multiple sclerosis have yet to be evaluated fully, but even now there is evidence that response to somatic stimulation of the limbs can be picked out from the cervical cord. If this observation

(Small *et al.* 1975) is confirmed there can be direct evidence of spinal cord involvement in demyelinating diseases.

The expectancy wave

The evoked response studies we have so far considered use runs of similar stimuli. In the experimental paradigm first reported by Grey Walter and colleagues in 1964 the method is different. The subject is presented with a warning stimulus, often a click delivered by earphones, which is then followed by another stimulus about a second later – a train of light flashes. The subject is instructed to respond when the flashes begin by pressing a switch which turns them off. In this experiment a negative wave appears between the warning stimulus and the flashes. The wave is only seen if the subject has been asked to respond to the flashes, and the moment the flashes are extinguished the wave disappears. Because the wave is contingent on the response, the term 'the Contingent Negative Variation' or CNV has been proposed and this is now the technical term rather than the more picturesque 'expectancy wave'. The CNV can sometimes be seen in the EEG without using a computer, but generally the responses to a set of pairs of stimuli are averaged so that they can be clearly delineated. The CNV can also be observed when other types of stimuli are used and other types of behavioural response required of the subject. It is not therefore dependent on motor action, a point of importance to which we shall return.

Of particular interest is the fact that the CNV is a brain response corresponding to a psychological process. Berger, the discoverer of the human EEG, was, as we have noted, a psychiatrist and must have been disappointed by the fact that the EEG did not seem to relate directly to mental function. The discovery of the CNV does appear to show that there is at least one direct relationship between brain activity and behaviour. As might be expected there are abnormalities in the CNV in various groups of psychiatric patients including the schizophrenic and the psychopathic (see Chapter 9).

The whole subject of the CNV has recently been reviewed (McCallum and Knott 1973), including some studies on changes found in organic brain disease. It has been shown, for example, that in patients with a cerebral tumour the CNV is suppressed over the site of the lesion. However, the place of this method in routine clinical work has yet to be assessed.

Computer assisted averaging techniques can also be used to delineate another type of small potential which is not a response to stimulation, but the precursor of motor movement. This so called 'readiness potential' (Kornhuber and Deecke 1965) is a slow negative wave seen over the rolandic region a second or so before the movement of the contralateral limb occurs. It is of great interest because it appears to be directly related to brain function and it could be regarded as the 'stimulus' for motor movement. The pre-motor potentials, however, are quite distinct from the CNV.

In conclusion, it is seen clearly that averaging techniques are an area of great intrinsic interest and, though in themselves they probably may have a limited overall contribution to the clinical field, they have acted as an impetus to clinical neurophysiology and have led to new ways of viewing and presenting cerebral potentials. They have brought to the fore the importance of techniques of quantification and data reduction and are really the first examples of computer technology to be directly applicable to clinical neurophysiological practice in the day-to-day hospital setting.

CHAPTER FOURTEEN

The EEG Report

The EEG request form and the report are usually the only channel of communication between the clinician and the electroencephalographer. This happens particularly where an EEG department may serve several hospitals and is unfortunate because misunderstandings can arise both in relation to referrals and in relation to the information furnished by the electroencephalographer. Often in these instances a telephone conversation can clarify the situation, either on the part of the clinician or on the part of the person reporting the EEG. In my own department I am able to see the majority of the people who use the EEG almost daily, because we work in a large teaching hospital and because the various offices and wards of referring doctors are situated close together. In addition there is opportunity, at least three times a week, to meet and discuss pathological, radiological and overall clinical problems currently under consideration. Nevertheless, difficulties do arise. Referral forms may be inadequately completed, or information may be omitted either by mistake or because it was not realised that it was important. Also, the electroencaphalographer may perhaps have failed to appreciate fully the problem, and his report as a result may be incomplete.

As with other types of investigation it is important to consider two separate aspects of the tests used: first, their reliability; and secondly, their validity (Rose *et al.* 1973).

Reliability as applied to electroencephalography would concern answers to such questions as: 'Would the EEG done on another occasion yield the same result?', 'Would the EEG report done by someone else be similar?', 'Would there be any agreement as to whether certain deflections were artefact or not?', 'Does the EEG show appropriate activity for drowsiness and sleep?', 'Does it contain sharp waves or spikes?'.

The simple answer to all these questions would be 'Yes', but this must be qualified by saying that differences do occur. Consider all the questions in relation to a patient with epilepsy. Variations between one record and the next may be due entirely to how recently a fit has occurred; if recently, it is more likely that the record will contain sharp waves and spikes. Drowsiness, also, is important, since it usually increases these abnormalities and may lead to differences between one EEG and the next on the same patient (Scott *et al.* 1974).

When it comes to deciding the types of phenomena seen, this can be solved in part by the use of inter-rater techniques. Such a method is particularly important in certain studies which we have carried out on hypnotics and tranquillising drugs (Malpas *et al.* 1970, Malpas *et al.* 1974). In a clinical situation it is also of significance (Scott *et al.* 1974), when we must try to determine whether the record is normal or abnormal. Clearly in research projects this is critical, but in the everyday clinical work of the department there is a strong case for suggesting that in the first instance the EEG should be looked through without reference either to the age of the patient or to the clinical information (Volavka *et al.* 1973). This 'blind' rating technique has in my view, been, under-employed. It sharpens the assessment and is a useful teaching vehicle. I do not suggest, however, that a report should be sent out without reading the request form since this would detract from the value of integrating EEG results into the whole clinical picture.

Quite often in teaching sessions we show a single page of an EEG recording and ask the questions: 'What is the age of the patient?', 'What is the state of consciousness?', 'What EEG phenomena are shown and what are their significance?'. It is interesting how frequently this intensive study of a single page of EEG may reveal unexpectedly large amounts of information. I shall return later to training in general.

Validity

Validity is a different concept from reliability. Validity concerns the meaning of the test in clinical terms, and this of course is of more significance to the referring doctor than the reliability. The doctor is interested in the individual patient referred on that particular occasion. It is therefore important that he should know what results to expect with a referral diagnosis of '?brain tumour'. He would expect a positive result for an intracerebral glioma, whereas the extracerebral meningioma may not reveal itself on the EEG. He should also be aware that one third to one half of EEGs on patients with infrequent generalised seizures may be quite normal. We shall return later to how we ourselves test out the accuracy of the reports.

EEG reporting

Reporting EEGs is a pattern-recognition task. Each person who does it has his own special way of carrying it out. However, in terms of economy of time, an initial quick run-through, scanning each page, is helpful. This will soon reveal whether there are many EEG phenomena to be examined or whether the whole of the tracing is rather similar; such an initial scanning contributes especially to a particular section of the EEG report, as I shall explain in a moment. In some departments it is customary for the technicians to carry out a detailed descriptive report on the EEG, and there the electroencephalographer may well read this and the clinical information – not only the information on the request form but additional information provided by the technician and usually written at the beginning of the EEG. On the whole, my view is that it is preferable to consider the EEG initially and rapidly, without reference to any additional information, not even the age of the patient, before making the detailed evaluation.

This first step in reporting includes a brief survey of artefact. The more detailed examination of this and other phenomena is reserved for the second stage. Then everything is assessed systematically – the type, amount, frequency, distribution of activity and so on. The state of the patient is taken into consideration and the neurological and other signs related to the phenomena seen. The patterns are matched with experience obtained in reporting thousands of EEGs previously – experience which covers a vast range of abnormal features and allows one to derive norms for particular ages.

I am often asked 'How does the process not become utterly boring?' The answer is that, partly because there is such an infinite variety in the patterns seen, one comes to recognise an EEG almost as that of a particular patient. The other factor to bear in mind is that the electroencephalographer, like the radiologist, often does see his patients. For example, there may be an epilepsy clinic run in conjunction with the EEG department. In any case, the electroencephalographer may be called to examine the patient because the technician cannot match her observations of the patient with what she sees in the EEG, or because the patient has a fit or appears to be in some curious mental state. In addition, he encounters the patient when undertaking special investigations such as a sphenoidal recording. Further, when patients are considered for surgery of epilepsy, the electroencephalographer is often asked not only to assess the EEGs but also to make some general comments on the suitability of the patient, comments which are taken into account by the surgeon in his final decision. The question of boredom relates obviously to motiviation (Scott 1970) and to a large extent to a subject's view of his value rather than to the specific task carried out.

The other question constantly asked is: 'How long does it take to report an EEG?' This is a difficult question to answer for it varies from a few minutes to perhaps an hour or more, depending on whether the record is routine and has very little in it or whether it is a complicated one containing many different phenomena and one on which a report for medico-legal purposes might have to be made. Length is a consideration here. Clearly the brief 15-minute routine recording takes less time to report than the hour-long tracing following oral barbiturate, and this does not approach the length of the 'all night' tracings carried out in the sleep laboratory.

Another question is: 'How long does it take to become an electroencephalographer, and what sort of training and background does he have?' The answer is that consultants at present have a wide variety of training and backgrounds, and there is some disagreement about what are the best prerequisites. Most encephalographers have a background of general medicine with neurology and psychiatry, and there are in addition a few non-medically qualified people with a scientific background who enter the field, usually in a research and academic capacity. The training must incorporate not only basic neurophysiology but also the physics and electronics necessary to understand electronic apparatus. As the field is rapidly developing and computers are used not only in a research capacity but also on day-to-day working basis, for example for evoked response studies, something of the basic technology here is essential. With all these prerequisites the ability to report EEG tracings is acquired relatively rapidly. After six months full-time in the field, a large proportion of recordings can be coped with, but as in other specialities a minimum time of two years as a senior registrar in a department of clinical neurophysiology having varied intake of different types of clinical material is essential before becoming a consultant.

The pattern-recognition techniques learnt in the process of training could be compared with those of an orchestral conductor in terms of the large amount of information which has to be scanned. There are, however, obvious differences, because in the EEG there is a considerable redundancy of information, as well as extraneous material that has to be eliminated from consideration, whereas one hopes this is not the situation with an orchestral score!

The EEG report

The EEG report is divided into two main sections (see Table 14.1). The first is largely factual and descriptive, and the second is an opinion of the significance of the tracing.

The first section of the report is again split into two parts. The first part is descriptive of the patient at the time of the EEG. If the patient had a seizure during the tracing itself, the clinical features seen would be described in detail – technicians have a considerable experience of seeing fits and often give very accurate accounts of what happened. If the

Table 14.1 The EEG report

Section 1

(a) State of patient at time of EEG. Description of seizures, etc., occurring during test.

(b) Factual report.
General description of EEG, e.g. markedly asymmetrical.
All normal and abnormal phenomena described in terms of frequency amplitude, site, symmetry, waveform and responsiveness, etc.
The effects of overbreathing and photic stimulation.

Section 2

(a) Summary of main EEG features.

(b) Possible clinical correlates.

(c) Any further EEG studies or other comments.

patient was unconscious the behavioural responses to stimulation would be noted. Sometimes the request form for an outpatient may be 'out of date' because the patient has had a seizure the night before the EEG. This is important to note because, like many of the other features mentioned in the first part of the report, it will have a direct bearing on the interpretation. Ordinarily, if the patient is alert and co-operative, this section of the report will be omitted.

The second part of this section is usually in a new paragraph, the first sentence of which will make some general statement about the EEG. The overall view gained by the first quick scanning by the electroencephalographer is here important. For example, 'The EEG is of low voltage and characterised by fast components' or 'The tracing is markedly asymmetrical' are the type of comments made.

Then follows a detailed analysis of the phenomena seen. The description is principally a record for the electroencephalographer so that, should the EEG not be available for direct comparison on a subsequent occasion, a statement can be made about differences between tracings. There are specific aspects of each EEG phenomenon which will be described. For example, frequency, amplitude, location, symmetry, wave form and responsiveness for all the features present will usually be given. There are also generally separate paragraphs for the effects of overbreathing and photic stimulation.

The second section – the opinion – can best be thought of as having three parts. The first part is a brief summary of the main EEG features: for example, the occurrence of temporal lobe sharp waves or a localised continuous frontal delta abnormality. The second puts forward the clinical correlate of the features seen. The third concerns any further action or suggestions in terms of EEG investigations. For example, if a patient presented with 'late onset epilepsy' and the EEG showed some localised features, then ordinarily it would be suggested that a further tracing be carried out in, say, three months' time. If the EEG showed only minor abnormalities in a patient in whom the diagnosis of epilepsy seemed likely but not certain, then a further tracing, for example with oral barbiturate, would be suggested. Sometimes the discrepancy between, say, the EEG features and the clinical history are impossible to reconcile. Then discussion with the clinician, either directly or by telephone, is indicated. This is also the course of action if, for example, a patient from a nearby psychiatric hospital shows a major localised abnormality which seems likely to require further investigation, or if the EEG of an infant has an hypsarrhymic pattern, a disturbance which generally means that urgent treatment is required. It is usual to record the clinical information and the EEG report on a card in the departmental files and to return the original to the clinician. This means that with subsequent referrals it is unnecessary for the initial clinical information to be repeated.

How we check our EEG reports against outcome

Another question often rightly asked is: 'How do you determine the accuracy of your reports in relation to the patient's final diagnosis?'

Basically we check our findings with the clinicians and with the neuro-radiologists and the physicists in the isotope brain scan department informally, as well as at meetings held at least weekly. In addition there is a weekly meeting with the neuro-pathologist at which biopsy results or neuro-pathological findings are discussed. Further, when serial recordings are carried out on patients, we have the benefit of updated clinical information as well as observations on the evolution of EEG features.

However, these methods, even taken together and carried out consistently and intensively, are still, in our view, inadequate for assessment of results. Therefore over the past ten years we have had a special EEG file on the hospital computer (Barber and Abbott 1972).

The development of a computer file

In the early 1960s it became apparent that a punch card system for collating EEG and clinical information was inadequate. As a result the computer file was established by my predecessor Dr. S.L. Last in 1964 (Krauthammer *et al.* 1966). At the present time some 25,000 records are on this file. This is not, it should be understood, raw EEG data, since this would present too large a 'data load' even for a large computer. The information on the EEG itself is therefore based on standardised visual ratings done at the time the tracing is reported.

Let us consider how the system works. The first stage depends on the EEG technician. She is responsible for filling in the patient's identification information on the first part of the input form, which we call a 'transcription sheet' (see Table 14.2). This she does when annotating the EEG recording and before taking it to the electroencephalographer for reporting. The encephalographer's first task is to check that the information has been filled in correctly. He then enters the diagnostic information and rings the other appropriate items. There are about 500 alternatives, which relate to the patient's clinical state, as well as the visual ratings of the various EEG phenomena seen (Tables 14.2, 3). They are thus stored in the computer file in a semi-quantitative fashion. The assessment is not as daunting as it sounds. After some practice it does not greatly add to the time taken for reporting the EEG.

When she types the report to the clinician, the department secretary checks that the transcription sheet has been adequately completed, and at least one item in each of the different boxes is ringed. The completed transcription sheets

Table 14.2

Patient information on the London Hospital transcription sheet used to input data into the EEG Computer file, and an example of one 'box' with EEG findings

CARD 1	EEG NO 2–6	Rep. 7–8	NAME 10–33	Hos. Code 34–35	Hospital No. 36–42
1					

AGE 43–45	SEX(M=1,F=2) 46	I.P.=1 or OP=2 47	REF. 48	DEPT. 49	TYPE OF REC. 50	DATE 51–58
						/ /

PROVISIONAL DIAGNOSIS 59–62	FINAL DIAGNOSIS (1) 63–65	FINAL DIAGNOSIS (2) 66–68	FINAL DIAGNOSIS (3) 69–71

Box 13

SPIKES AND SHARP WAVES

Present	360
Overbreathing only	361
Photic stimulation only	362
Single many	363
Single few	364
Dubious	365
Groups	366
Localised	367
Several foci	368
Mirror foci	369
Occipital spikes	370
Not localised	371
Subclinical seizure discharge	372
Appears or increases with drowsiness and sleep	373
None	399

are then despatched to the computer department at weekly intervals. There the transcription sheets are punched on to cards. Part of the computer program involves checks and validates the cards as the data are entered into the computer file. If errors are found, the record is rejected and an error report printed. This is then returned to the EEG department for correction.

The transcription sheet (see Table 14.2) is divided into sub-sections. Apart from the obvious identification of the patient, we also have information relating to the referral department, so that we can check who our main users are. These figures were presented in Chapter 1, indicating, for example, that 30% of our referrals are from neurologists and 15% from paediatricians.

We also have a code number which indicates what type of EEG recording was carried out. Thus if special techniques were used, or if it was a tracing carried out in the ward, this is noted. It is useful information in planning, in terms both of work load and of space and staff requirements for the future.

The second part of the sheet is the diagnostic section (Table 14.2). There are four sub-divisions: one for 'provisional diagnosis' and three for 'final diagnoses'. Our diagnostic index has been built up over the years, and each doctor reporting EEGs has a copy on his desk. The third part of the sheet consists of 22 boxes to be filled in for most EEGs. The first three refer to the state of the patient and any procedures carried out during the tracing. The next group relates to EEG features, both general and specific. The information entered on the sheet is descriptive, as well as semi-quantitative. For example, 'spikes single/few', item 264 (see table 14.2) means isolated spikes or sharp waves, less than 10 in the whole of the EEG. The definitions we use for many of these items are based on international conventions, but we have extended the range of these considerably (see Glossary). A copy of the definitions is available on the electroencephalographer's desk, so that he can refresh his memory of them if necessary. The fact that we have definitions of many EEG features and a standardised transcription sheet is particularly useful when a new member of staff is appointed to the department. He learns a standard way of making an EEG report based on a more logical assessment of features seen. Further, by close adherence to these definitions he will learn to use terms correctly and with precision and increase inter-rater reliability (Volavka *et al.* 1973). This is one advantage of the particular system.

Further, we have an amendment sheet, so that when other information accrues during the patient's stay in hospital – for example, more accurate diagnostic information from neuro-radiological studies, from isotope brain scanning or as a result of neurosurgical operation – this can be added to the patient's file (Table 14.3). Later, we may wish to code the fact that the patient died and that autopsy information is available. The ability to up-date the information on the file – and this can be done a number of times for each patient – is of particular importance when we are carrying out retrospective investigations to verify the EEG reports previously made.

There are two main types of computer program used to search the EEG file. The first is for 'housekeeping'. The up-to-date file is searched and each record checked to see whether it falls within a specific date range. The resulting group of records is then analysed by type, range, referral department, etc., and the overall total is printed out. We obtain such a print-out quarterly and annually. This indicates the total work load and how it is distributed, in terms of both the type of records and of referral departments. We can also see how many long and complicated records have been carried out. By comparison with the work in previous years, it is possible to determine what areas show a markedly increased work load, and thus we can make more accurate predictions about expansion of facilities.

The second type of computer program is the 'search program'. This allows us to have easy and rapid access to the data stored. We can find out how many patients we have on the file with a particular diagnosis or combination of diagnoses; for example, both migraine and epilepsy. This was important a few years ago when we were beginning a programme on the investigation of these conditions. We knew immediately that 157 patients had been seen with that dual diagnosis over the previous ten years. The figure proved fairly

Table 14.3 Two 'boxes' on London Hospital Computer sheet, one for information on clinical localisation and the other a summary of EEG information and findings of special investigations

Box 21
CLINICAL LOCALISATION

Known	900
Unknown	901
Single	902
Multiple	903
One sided	904
Bilateral	905
Left frontal	906
Right frontal	907
Left temporal	908
Right temporal	909
Left parietal	910
Right parietal	911
Left occipital	912
Right occipital	913
Parasagittal	914
Anterior cranial fossa	915
Middle cranial fossa	916
Posterior cranial fossa	917
Corpus callosum	918
Rolandic	919
Optic nerve and chiasma	920
Sphenoidal ridge	921
Third ventricle	922
Sylvian	923
Thalamus	924
Subcortical	925
Basal ganglia	926
Cerebellum	927
Mid brain	928
Pons	929
Brain stem	930
Left (overall lateralisation)	931
Right (overall lateralisation)	932
Cervical spine	933
None	949

Box 22
SUMMARY

Normal	950
Doubtful	951
Mildly abnormal	952
Moderately abnormal	953
Severely abnormal	954
Record improved	955
Record deteriorated	956
Clinical diagnosis (final)	966
Laboratory (biochemistry etc).	967
Scan (isotope)	968
Neuroradiology	969
Biopsy confirmation	970
Patient now dead	971
P.M. performed	972

accurate, because we were able to investigate ten such patients in a prospective way over the following year. Another example was as follows. A patient with chronic renal failure, undergoing regular dialysis, unexpectedly had an epileptic fit. The EEG was markedly abnormal, and we were uncertain whether this was the result of her renal condition or indicative of some independent cerebral lesion such as a tumour. A rapid print-out of patients with renal failure was obtained, which indicated that the EEG features our patient showed were quite unlike those of the 170 cases on the file. This was reported to the clinician in question, and careful consultation with other hospitals which the patient had attended before revealed that she had a benign cerebral vascular malformation detected some years previously, which was presumably the cause of the fit.

Using a search program, we were able to determine the particular type of EEG abnormality and the severity of this for any particular diagnosis. This is especially important because selection factors operate strongly in EEG work, and as a result the findings reported by other workers may not be directly applicable to our own data. Let us take an example – a section of a computer print-out of fact 106 (as seen in Table 14.4), the number which corresponds to bifrontal delta activity. From the print-out we were able to determine that, in the group of patients in whom it occurred, 79% had intracranial lesions; but it was found that about 10% had systemic disturbance leading to secondary brain dysfunction. It thus confirmed our clinical hunch, which was markedly at variance with published findings (for example, Cordeau 1959), and showed that particular care must be taken in the interpretation of EEGs in which bifrontal delta occurs.

The computer file was used to search for suitable patient material in studies of EEG changes with hyperventilation (Morgan and Scott 1970), those due to hypo- and hypercalcaemia (Swash and Rowan 1972), on temporal lobe epilepsy (Currie *et al.* 1971) and with cerebral metastases (Rowan *et al.* 1974). These projects have been completed, but others are in process of data collection. For example, a new diagnostic number has recently been assigned for epileptic patients having EEGs to determine whether or not anti-convulsants should be withdrawn. In the follow-up period, say in five years, it will be possible to determine whether the EEG features seen gave an indication of which patients would relapse if anticonvulsants were withdrawn.

A file of this kind is not the only use of computers in the EEG department. In the long run their main application is for signal analysis, and we shall find in Chapter 15 that results of this are already beginning to emerge. Nevertheless, the computer file is a great help in routine work, allowing us to

Table 14.4 Section of computer printout; see text for details

NAME		EEG NO.	HOSP. NO.	D.1.	D.2.	DATE	FACTS								
S	E	1671100	0	239	185		53	59	63	65	75	78	81	98	104
							105	106	142	152	154	182			
P	J	1673800	3571855	165	307		53	56	63	65	75	78	91	92	103
							106	142	151	152	154	155	182		
F	G	1675200	365149	165		7	55	56	63	65	75	77	78	91	101
							106	140	152	182					
E	T	1677200	0	1171		67	11	52	56	63	65	73	74	75	77
							78	81	91	92	94	97	102	106	108
L	W	1679900	370511	167		/67	141	142	151	154	155	156	157	182	
							11	52	56	63	65	71	76	78	81
B	F	1680600	370516	8		11/67	91	92	103	106	108	140	151	152	154
							155	156	157	182					
							53	59	63	65	72	75	78	81	91
							92	94	97	104	106	134	142	152	154
							155	182							
P	C	1683300	0			/11/67	53	56	63	65	77	78	81	91	102
							106	142	144	151	152	154	182	194	
P	C	1683302	0			/12/67	53	56	63	65	75	78	81	91	101
							106	142	151	154	182				
T	F	1689300	370190			14/12/67	55	56	63	65	71	74	77	78	91
							97	101	103	106	108	141	142	151	152
							182								

have access to a much larger 'experience' than would be possible using our memories and individual files of 'interesting cases'.

In conclusion, it can be seen that the EEG report has a precise format. Furthermore, electroencephalographers are aware of the limitation of the reports and endeavour by a variety of means to check and improve accuracy. It is also possible to quantify visual ratings of EEG in a way that allows them to aid clinical research projects. This relatively simple technique should be much more widely applied, and the methods are useful in a whole range of biological data collected and collated in hospital practice.

CHAPTER FIFTEEN

The Problems and Future of EEG

The fact that the EEG was first reported to the world as recently as 1929 emphasises that it is still a relatively young subject. In human terms, therefore, the present period may be seen, not only as a time for consolidation, but also as one for developing new ideas with the maturity of middle age rather than the heady enthusiasm of youth. Nevertheless, clinical electroencephalography has certainly had its share of critics, including recently Matthews (1973) and Pappworth (1974). No one would deny that there are problems. Let us see how they arise and in what ways they may be resolved in the not too distant future. We shall later consider also some recent advances in the field.

A basic problem

The EEG is performed with a limited number of electrodes, about 20, each usually one centimetre in diameter, placed 3½ to 4 centimetres apart in a symmetrical fashion on the scalp. Any particular electrode is influenced by a cone-shaped area of brain cells. This is explained by the so-called 'shadowing theorem'. We imagine an electric light bulb above the head casting a shadow of the electrode, say six centimetres in diameter, on the surface of the cortex. Of course, between the electrode and the cortical surface there is a barrier of tissue which has an averaging and damping effect. As we know from direct cortical recording in the operating theatre, a fivefold overall attentuation of potentials occurs. However, a localised spike on the cortical surface may appear in the scalp recording as a sharp wave; that is, a potential of longer duration and of markedly diminished amplitude. Indeed attentuation of individual cortical spikes can be as great as by a factor of a hundred (Goldensohn *et al.* 1970). How many cells, in fact, are responsible for the alpha rhythm? MacGillivray (1974) suggested that each cell could be regarded as producing a potential of a hundredth of a microvolt. To lead to an alpha rhythm of a hundred microvolts we would assume that a hundred thousand cells would be involved. Considering the configuration of the cortical surface it would be realised that only the cells at the tips of gyri would be contributing to the recorded EEG, while those at right angles and buried in the depths of the sulci are unlikely to contribute greatly. It is interesting, however, that only in rare instances is it worth using extra electrodes, say 1½ to 2 centimetres apart. This particular instance is when the patient is having a Jacksonian attack and the ordinary recording does not show any discharge. Because closer spacing of electrodes rarely yields further information we naturally assume that, although the cortical cells themselves are responsible for the scalp EEG, the deeper connections with mid-line structures, in particular thalamus and the reticular formation, have an influence on a wider area of cortical cells (see Chapter 2). Then a number of electrodes and several channels of the recording are usually involved in the disturbance.

If the total head of electrodes is considered, it will be realised that they are relatively remote from large areas of cortex, especially the under folded temporal lobes, which comprise as much as a sixth of all the cortex. Thus, taking all these factors into consideration, McGillivray estimated that the EEG represents a sampling of perhaps a third of 1% of all brain cells, a view which goes some way to explaining why, for example, a normal EEG may be found in a patient with epilepsy. Perhaps it is surprising that we have so many positive results!

Technical difficulties

It is clear that there are technical difficulties too. Those are dealt with elsewhere (Cooper *et al.* 1974). One striking example is as follows. The ordinary EEG electrode is made of silver with a soldered copper wire attached. If a pair of these electrodes is placed in a bath of saline, the ordinary conducting medium for the recording, and attached to a measuring device, they lead to voltages far in excess of genuine brain potentials. This is just one of the problems that has to be overcome by the design of the EEG recording system. Another is the ubiquitous 50-cycle-per-second impulses emanating from electrical apparatus in the region of the EEG machine. Without appropriate rejection factors, again part of the design of the apparatus, the tracings would be completely masked and uninterpretable.

Personnel

The personnel carrying out the tracings are either the weakest link in the chain or the strongest, depending on how they have been trained. They have many functions. The first is to put the patient at his ease, so that muscle artefact, eye blink and other biological but non-brain potentials which mask the cortical activity are reduced to a minimum. The second is to recognise the patterns which are emerging as the tracing proceeds. Are these from the brain? Are they from the electrode? Are they from outside interference? The technician must correct the apparatus or make adjustments to the electrodes during the recording itself, as well as selecting appropriate electrode linkages to display the brain activity most effectively. Once the recording has been completed and the electrodes removed, nothing can be done with a technically poor EEG except to repeat it.

EEG interpretation and quantification

Reporting the EEG (see Chapter 14) presents a number of difficulties, and perhaps the first is who should do it. Should it be the technician or a medically trained person? Unfortunately, in my view, in many centres the technicians are virtually responsible for the interpretation and for a number of reasons medical supervision is scanty. This has two implications. First, the standard of recordings tends to deteriorate unless correctible artefacts are pointed out to the technician at the time of the recording or as soon after as is possible. Secondly, it means that the EEG technicians are sometimes giving reports direct to clinicians without the intervention of an electroencephalographer. Such a procedure can only lead to difficulties, since a great number of technicians may not have experience of the clinical significance of particular findings and may not appreciate all their implications. This can only lead to denigration of EEG.

The next problem is: what does the EEG actually contain? Apart from brain potentials, a whole series of other deflections are seen, as we have already noted (see Chapter 2). Many of these artefacts may mimic cerebral activity but are not from the brain at all. Here it is only by experience that the electroencephalographer can sort out the 'wheat from the tares'. In addition, accurate definition of the various types of brain potentials is essential. These have been decided at an international level for general EEG phenomena (Chatrian *et al.* 1974) and for sleep changes in detail (Rechschaften and Kales 1969). Further, we ourselves have found value in a series of departmental definitions which run into several hundreds of items, covering almost all types of important EEG phenomena. They are of particular importance in relation to our EEG computer file (Chapter 14), allowing consistent filling-in of data sheets sent to the computer department.

Another aspect of EEG interpretation concerns the subjective element and how it may be reduced. I have already mentioned a simple approach which is applicable in day-to-day work: to look at the EEG before studying the request form (see Chapter 14). However, there are other more complex approaches which are mainly applicable to research. The EEGs can be masked and coded, so that the phenomena can not only be identified but also quantified without reference to anything other than previously decided information, for example the age of the patient. In addition more than one rater can study the tracings independently, and discussion can take place on points of difference between the ratings. Surprisingly enough, when definitions have been well drawn up it is possible to learn relatively rapidly techniques of quantification, by 'eyeballing', so that results are reducible from occasion to occasion and there is also agreement between individuals.

In previous chapters I have indicated where quantification of the EEG by eye is not only possible but extremely valuable, for example in the assessment of the EEG changes following cerebral anoxia, as well as in patients with cerebral metastases, to give two clinical examples. It can also be of help in detecting patients taking barbiturates illicitly (West and Driver 1974). In the more research-orientated sphere it helps the assessment of hypnotic drugs and the investigation of various sleep disorders using all-night sleep recordings (see Chapter 10). In addition compressed EEG records produced by the Cerebral Function Monitor (Schwartz *et al.* 1972) are also amenable to direct measurement as well as evoked responses from stimulation by light or sound.

Having obtained numerical data from EEG, the next and final stage, the relationship between it and the clinical outcome, can more readily be assessed. It has proved possible in relation to both the clinical examples I have cited, cerebral anoxia and cerebral matastases (Prior 1973, Rowan *et al.* 1974). In this final stage of matching the EEG findings to the final diagnosis, the EEG computer file has been extremely valuable since it is possible to add subsequent clinical, pathological or other types of information to the patient's EEG data, and when retrospective studies are carried out the data are readily available directly from a computer print-out.

Advantages of EEG

In spite of the problems at various levels that I have described in detail, EEG requests are increasing every year, and on this ground alone it does appear that clinicians find value in the investigation. Among its advantages (see Table 15.1) is the fact that it is a non-invasive test which can be repeated readily – if there is a question of a cerebral abscess for example, even at daily intervals, and in patients in whom there is a question of 'brain death' the recording can be repeated in 12 hours. When the provisional diagnosis is late-onset epilepsy and there seems likely to be an underlying structural lesion, then 3-monthly or 6-monthly repeats can be arranged. The same applies after head injury, to check the progress and possibly detect the emergence of discrete 'epileptic' activity

Table 15.1 The problems and advantages of EEG

Problems	*Advantages*
Remoteness of electrodes from some brain areas	Non-invasive
Technical problems	Can be repeated frequently
Personnel recruitment and training	Relatively cheap
EEG interpretation and validation	Shows CNS dysfuntion as well as structural abnormality

of the type already mentioned (Chapter 7), features which preceded the development of epilepsy in patients with treated cerebral abscess. The EEG is innocuous from the patient's point of view, and it is relatively cheap compared with other investigations of the central nervous system. It costs in the region of £20, perhaps half the cost of radio-isotope brain scan. Whether the EMI scan will be cheaper is uncertain, but the capital outlay for EEG equipment is between £5,000 and £10,000, which is only the fraction of the capital cost of the computer-assisted-tomography-of-the-head apparatus. We will not dwell on the research uses of EEG already mentioned in passing, but I wish to underline the clinical applications of electroencephalography. In particular it is of value for patients with structural lesions, cerebral tumours, cerebral abscess and cerebrovascular accidents. Of equal or perhaps great importance is its use in 'dysfunctional' processes, the major example of which is epilepsy. Even if its value is to some extent usurped by the EMI scanner, in patients with structural disease the use in the investigation of epilepsy will continue.

The EEG has been utilised in a wide variety of conditions, including simulated unconsciousness (Hopkins 1973) and transient global amnesia (Croft *et al.* 1973), in neurosurgical practice in the location of a bleeding aneurysm (Margerison *et al.* 1969) especially where there are multiple aneurysms and on clinical or other grounds it is unclear which has ruptured. Schwartz *et al.* (1973) have employed EEG in a compressed form to predict clinical outcome after cardiac surgery, and it has been used to monitor cerebral perfusion during internal carotid surgery (Editorial 1974).

Investigation of delirium following surgical operations is also currently under investigation using EEG techniques (Johns *et al.* 1974) as well as in the assessment of patients with fulminating hepatic failure (Gazzard *et al.* 1974).

EEG signal analysis

So far in this book I have concentrated largely on interpretation of the EEG record by visual inspection and the recognition of common patterns. This technique is universally used because of the relative ease with which EEGs can be obtained, interpreted and permanently recorded. Admittedly this last presents storage problems because of bulk, but the technology of the ink-written trace is relatively straightforward. I have already mentioned two other methods of dealing with EEG data. First of all there is the obtaining of a write-out of the frequency content using a so-called 'frequency analyser' (see Chapter 8). This apparatus produces histograms of frequencies in the EEG for every ten seconds of actual recording. It has been used to determine changes with age and alterations following the administration of drugs, as well as for the assessment of hemispheric asymmetries of activity. However, information about the actual wave-form of the EEG components is lost by this technique. There is another different approach, namely the study of responses following stimulation – averaged evoked responses. Here, a train of stimuli are presented and averaged using a small pre-programmed computer (see Chapter 13). This has advantages in terms of data reduction and also the wave-form obtained can be measured simply by a ruler. Unfortunately variability, which may be significant from a physiological or pathological point of view over a particular run of stimuli, is lost. Both frequency analysis and evoked response techniques allow quantification and add a new dimension to EEG analysis. Both of these are now available for routine clinical use although unfortunately not every department has access to them at present.

These, however, are not the only techniques currently of interest. There are others which employ medium-sized and large computers able to cope with the data load presented by the EEG. The signals can be analysed, and not just in terms of frequency or amplitude: the wave-form can also be taken into consideration. Moreover, there is a great variety of ways in which the processed signals can be presented (see for example Kellaway and Petersen 1973). It is beginning to be possible to delinineate series of waves which form a pattern characteristic of a particular condition. The simplest is the spike-and-wave complex seen in patients with petit mal epilepsy. Using large computers it is easy to specify limits of variability in the relationship of the various components one with another. The EEG can also be recorded on tape and processed repeatedly, searches being made successively for different wave-forms or other features. Other techniques have also been adopted using computers. It is possible to display brain activity in the form of a 'contour map,' but instead of height above sea level and distance as parameters, time and potential changes are used (see, for example, Maynard 1972). At a recent EEG Society meeting in Edinburgh (Johnson *et al.* 1975) there was considerable discussion about the many recent advances in computer technology and its application to clinical electroencephalography. Great interest was expressed, and it was felt that, even within the next five years, there might be great progress in their use in routine work. This certainly offers at the very least a means of reduction of the subjective element in EEG assessment. However, it is still necessary for the findings to be related to the clinical features and outcome. Here liaison between the electroencephalographer and his clinical colleagues will still be of great importance.

Telemetry

The application of large computers to the analysis of EEG is not the only advance in the field. One important new technique is telemetry. This, though possible for several years, is now beginning to have an impact in ordinary clinical work. The principle is simple, though the technology is somewhat involved. Basically, biological signals are converted into radio waves and transmitted from the human or animal, to be received at a distance and in many instances written out in the usual way as an ink-on-paper trace. However, there are no intervening wires, and the technique allows a whole new range of studies to be undertaken.

The principle has been applied in 3 main ways (Wolff 1967). The first is the so-called 'radio pill' which, after being swallowed by the patient, broadcasts the state of his gastro-intensinal tract, its mobility and acidity. The second, which applies to EEG work, is somewhat different. The freely moving patient carries on his person apparatus which transmits his EEG for a distance of up to about 100 yards. The signal can be picked by an aerial and recorded or written out. The third type of telemetry came about during the space programme. Here ECG and even EEG were transmitted through space to be received 'on earth'.

Obviously telemetry has implications in research, but from a clinical point of view it has two special uses: first of all in children, particularly those who are behaviourally disturbed, and secondly in patients with epilepsy. In both instances the patients can be under study while carrying out relatively normal tasks in the hospital environment. For the subject with epilepsy, observation of seizure frequency can be carried out by a special nurse, or a video-tape monitor can be used. This has the advantage that the tape can be subsequently compared with the EEG tracing and the number of discharges compared with the obvious behavioural seizures. The recording can also be continued during sleep. Clearly this technique is time-consuming and the data accumulated are voluminous, and so only a relatively small number of patients can be studied intensively. One ingenious method to cope with this is being attempted. The EEG transmission and recording takes place only when a seizure discharge occurs. As the seizures are of high amplitude they can be used to trigger the recording system. In this way the amount of data collected is markedly reduced and is thus more manageable from the point of view of subsequent analysis.

Early results from the studies on epileptic patients (Stevens *et al.* 1971, Geier 1971) show that EEG discharges are more frequent than overt seizures. Further, there is an interesting and marked diurnal-nocturnal variation in the occurrence of discharges. It appears that telemetry will be an extremely useful adjunct to the detection and management of seizures in difficult cases and also in the testing of the therapeutic regime in some subjects with intractable epilepsy.

Biofeedback

Biofeedback is another quite different recent advance sometimes involving electroencephalographic techniques. In a general context, it results from the experiments by the American psychologist Neil Miller. In essence it is simple. Electronic instruments are used to measure physiological parameters, such as blood pressure and EEG, and the information is immediately presented to the patient in the form either of a visual display or a tone of variable pitch. He learns as a result of the 'feedback' to exert a degree of control over a physiological process which would be quite impossible unless he was immediately aware of any change at the moment it occurred. From the EEG point of view the main interest has been in 'alpha machines'. These are simple and relatively cheap devices which tell the subject, usually by means of a tone of variable pitch or intensity, the state of his alpha rhythm. This has a therapeutic application based on the observation that relaxed subjects show well-sustained high-voltage alpha activity while tense and anxious individuals show very little. Thus, the individual learns to increase his alpha output, and this leads to relaxation and apparently to a sense of increased well-being. So far, although the field is one of 'explosive' interest, relatively few well-controlled studies have been carried out. Whether it is a really effective therapy remains to be seen, but it offers new possibilities in the treatment of a whole variety of psychosomatic disorders.

Epilepsy is one condition in which attempts have been made to use biofeedback. Some patients, in spite of apparent adequate anticonvulsant medication, fail to have satisfactory control of seizures, and Sterman and colleagues (for example, Sterman *et al.* 1974) have in such patients reported some success. We ourselves (Cabral and Scott 1975) have studied similar patients, attempting to compare the effect of relaxation (a modification of the Jacobsen technique) with a biofeedback method, in which the patient is taught to control the alpha rhythm and increase its amount. Preliminary results indicate that both techniques are effective in a small group of patients, though there is a suggestion that biofeedback may be more effective.

Conclusion

It is clear from this account that electroencephalography has a wide application in the field of clinical medicine and also in research. There are, apart from the routine techniques, interesting new advances in many directions. It is a subject which demands to be understood in order to be used properly, and I hope my account of what goes on in the EEG department and what can and cannot be expected from electroencephalography has gone some way to alleviate problems of communication and misunderstanding which have arisen in the past between electroencephalographers and their clinical colleagues.

Glossary

This glossary has been compiled over the years, mainly in the course of teaching those encountering EEG for the first time. It is intended to serve as a starting-point for discussion and study. Many of the definitions are those used for coding data on the London Hospital computer transcription sheet (see Chapter 14). The list is based on the various published glossaries of the International Federation of Societies of Electroencephalography and Clinical Neurophysiology, including the most recent (Chatrian, G.E., Bergamini, I.L., Dondey, M.O., Klass, D.W., Lennox-Buchthal, M. and Petersen, I., 1974, 'A glossary of terms most commonly used by clinical electroencephalographers', *Electroencephalography and Clinical Neurophysiology, 37,* 538). I am grateful to have been able to benefit from the hard work of these committees, and the many ideas they have put forward.

Abundance	Quantity of activity.
Active electrode	Synonym for exploring electrode. Any electrode intended to detect EEG activity input into 'black' lead (q.v.).
Active sleep	Neonatal sleep pattern equivalent to the REM sleep of adults (q.v.).
Activity	Any sequence of waves.
Activation	Any procedure which changes the EEG or enhances abnormality; for example, hyperventilation is used to elicit spike and wave in petit mal patients.
All night sleep recordings	EEG done with the purpose of ascertaining the amount of REM or paradoxical sleep occurring. Often used for the assessment of hypnotic drugs.

Alpha coma	Rare condition in which the EEG is dominated by alpha frequency activity which is unusually monotonous and widespread and shows no response to any form of stimulus. This occurs in deeply comatose patients and may be associated with pontine lesions.
Alpha rhythm	Seen in the alert adult subject with a frequency of 8 to 13½ cycles per second. It is most prominent over the posterior areas, present when the eyes are closed, and attentuated during attention, especially visual.
Amplitude	Voltage of EEG waves, usually expressed in microvolts peak to peak.
Analysers	See Frequency analyser.
Array	An arrangement of scalp electrodes.
Artefact	Any deflection in the recording arising either from the electrodes, or the apparatus, or from extracranial structures, such as the temporalis muscles or the eyes.
Asymmetry	Differences between the hemispheres for any activity, in terms of amplitude, amount and frequency. It may be of physiological or pathological significance.
Atrophic lesions	Lesions leading to diminution of background activities in general, though fast components may sometimes be augmented over the area in question.
Attenuation	Reduction of EEG activity; for example, of alpha rhythm when the eyes are opened.
Averaging	Shortened term for the technique used

to demonstrate 'Averaged evoked responses'. A computer-assisted method for displaying small responses resulting from cortical stimulation, e.g. visual.

Average reference recording	Method of referential recording in which the algebraic sum of potentials from all scalp electrodes acts as an 'indifferent' source, i.e. is fed into the 'white' lead (q.v.).
Background activity	Term used for the dominant activity in a particular region.
Beta activity	Term used to indicate waves or a rhythm with a frequency of 14 cycles per second or higher. Each wave will have a period of 1/14th of a second or less. Beta activity is present in most adult records over the anterior head regions and is prominent in patients receiving such drugs as barbiturate, when it is usually at 20–24 cycles per second.
Bilateral	Occurring on both sides of the head.
Bilateral synchrony	A term used to describe an EEG phenomenon – spike and wave – which occurs over both hemispheres at the same time. Generally it is a form of centrencephalic epilepsy, for example petit mal or grand mal. In rare instances it may be the result of a focal cortical process, when the term 'secondary bilateral synchrony' is given.
Bipolar recording	Here the active and indifferent electrodes or 'black' and 'white' leads are both attached to 'active' scalp electrodes. This may give rise to some difficulties, and the recording is best

	considered in relation either to common average reference or common reference recording.
Black lead	Active input to the amplifying system of each channel, so arranged that a negative potential causes an upward deflection.
Blocking	Term used to describe the attenuation of the alpha activity when the eyes are opened or other mental 'activity' occurs.
Burst	Group of waves which appear and disappear and are distinguished from the background by differences of frequency, form and amplitude.
Burst-suppression	Pattern in which episodes of activity are followed by periods when the EEG is isoelectric or nearly so. Seen in a variety of conditions including deep anaesthesia and severe anoxic cerebral insults.
Calibration	System of detailed checks (see Chapter 1) carried out to ensure that each channel of the EEG apparatus is behaving in a similar fashion in terms both of size of deflection and of its other characteristics.
Carotid compression	Technique used to test the integrity of cerebral vessels. The EEG is monitored during compression to see if abnormality appears.
Centrencephalic epilepsy	Epilepsy which arises as a result of a disturbance in mid-line structures often with a genetic component. It leads to generalised EEG discharge, for example, in grand mal or petit mal;

	contrast focal cortical epilepsy (see Chapter 4).
Cerebral function monitor (CFM)	Simple device used to obtain a compressed EEG record over long periods; for example, during cardiac surgery.
Channel	System for the detection, amplification and display of potential differences between a pair of electrodes. Usually an EEG machine has eight or more channels each acting simultaneously and independently.
CNV	Short for 'contingent negative variation', and often called the 'expectancy wave'. It appears in the EEG when the subject has heard a warning stimulus and is prepared to respond in a specific manner to the next stimulus (see Chapter 13).
Common mode rejection	Characteristic of the amplifiers used in EEG machines, the so-called differential amplifiers. Any signal which is common to the two imput terminals is rejected whereas signals which are different are amplified (see Discrimination).
Common reference	Accepted term for 'monopolar recording' (q.v.).
Complex	Group of two or more waves, clearly distinguished from background activity, occurring with a well-recognised form or recurring with consistent form, e.g. spike and wave complexes. They may be localised or generalised.
Convention, EEG	Convention indicating the direction of pen deflection depending on the polarity of the signals applied to the

	'black' and 'white' leads. If a negative potential is applied to the 'black' lead the pen deflection is upwards.
Corticography	Short for 'electrocorticography' (ECoG).
Cycle	Complete series of potential changes undergone by a wave before the same series is repeated.
Cycles per second	Abbreviation: c/sec. Equivalent to Herz per second – abbreviation, Hz/sec.
Delta	Used to indicate waves or rhythms in the resting record with a frequency of four cycles per second or less. Each wave has a period of a quarter of a second or more.
Delta, bifrontal	Bursts of sinusoidal waves at approximately two cycles per second, occurring abruptly bilaterally and bisynchronously and maximally in the frontal leads; synonymous with monorhythmic frontal delta. It implies dysfunction and is a form of 'rhythm at a distance'.
Delta, local	Such activity, if continuous and affecting two or three electrodes, implies localised structural damage.
Delta, posterior temporal	Isolated delta waves seen in the temporal leads of the EEGs of children or adolescents or 'immature' adults, disappearing when the eyes are open.
Depth EEG	Recording from electrodes inserted into the brain substance by the neurosurgeon. This can take place at the time of operation, though electrodes may be left in for days or weeks. Used to locate the site of a seizure discharge.

Derivation	Recording from a pair of electrodes or leads, the output of which is displayed on one channel of the tracing.
Differential amplifier	Amplifier whose output is proportional to the voltage difference between the two input terminals.
Diffuse	Occurring over large areas without constant location; compare Random.
Diphasic wave	Wave with two components, one on either side of the baseline; synonym, 'biphasic'.
Dipole	Electrical 'unit' having equal and opposite voltages separated in space. Used to facilitate theoretical discussion about the electrical fields on and around the brain surface.
Discharge	Sudden disturbance in the EEG often of spikes, sharp waves or slow components, either localised or generalised, usually signifying epilepsy.
Discontinuous	The alert adult shows cerebral activity which is continuous. In contrast the neonate, or the anaesthetised or the unconscious adult patient may show discontinuous activity, i.e. burst-suppression (q.v.).
Discrimination	Ability of the EEG machine to discriminate biological (out-of-phase) and non-biological (in-phase) signals so that the output is truly representative of cerebral activity (see Common mode rejection).
Discrimination ratio	Mathematical relationships between the in-phase and out-of-phase signals rejected by the EEG machine. Often of the order of 10,000 to 1.

Disorganised	Used to describe an EEG in which there is a combination of many types of activity with varying amplitude and frequency; synonym, 'irregular'.
Dominant	Frequency which characterises the EEG, usually taken to relate to the posterior part of the head. It would be 9 to 10 cycles per second for a normal adult.
Dysfunction	Disturbance seen in an EEG which does not necessarily imply a structural 'lesion' in the area over which the disturbance is seen.
Dysrhythmic	Abnormal EEG pattern. There is no general agreement on the features constituting it, and so the term is not recommended.
Electrical silence	No electrical activity (see Isoelectric EEG).
Electro-corticogram	Record of EEG activity obtained by means of leads directly applied over or inserted into the cerebral cortex; abbreviation 'ECoG'.
Electrode resistance	Measure of the opposition to flow of a current between the EEG electrode and the scalp or brain. It is tested between a pair of electrodes. In practical terms, if the scalp-electrode contact is poor, the tracing is technically sub-standard.
Electro-encephalogram	Record of electrical activity of the brain taken by means of electrodes placed on the scalp.
Electro-encephalograph	Instrument used to record electro-encephalograms.

Epileptic pattern	See Epileptiform pattern.
Epileptiform pattern	Distinctive pattern of waves or complexes easily distinguished from background activity, usually spikes and sharp waves (q.v.) but may be complexes. They are seen in the inter-ictal records of epileptic patients. Contrast Seizure discharge.
Episode	See Paroxysm.
Epoch	Period of time in the EEG recording arbitrarily determined for assessment either visually or automatically; for example, by means of a frequency analyser. Often a period of ten seconds is chosen.
Equipotential	Used to describe regions of the head or electrodes which are at the same potential at a given time. Hence the output from an amplifier attached to two electrodes in an equipotential region will on bipolar recording show no pen deflection; contrast monopolar recording.
Evoked response or potential	Cortical activity resulting from, for example, visual auditory or other stimuli. The waves may be small and not seen in the conventional EEG; hence an 'averaging' computer is used. In essence, it adds up the responses and eliminates the on-going EEG.
Expectancy wave	See CNV.
Fast activity	Activity of a higher frequency than alpha; that is, beta activity (q.v.).
Flat EEG	Term best avoided as it may lead to confusion between a low voltage record and one devoid of cerebral

	activity, i.e. the isoelectric tracing (q.v.).
Flattening	Term used rather losely, implying either disease in the cortex itself leading to diminution of recorded activity or something between the brain and the recording electrodes for example, a subdural haematoma.
Filters	EEG apparatus is fitted with two types of filter, the high frequency filters, which attenuate high frequency elements, particular muscle artefacts, and the low frequency filter which reduces slow components.
FIRDA	See Frontal Intermittent Rhythmic Delta Activity.
Focal cortical epilepsy	Condition in which seizures commence in a localised area of cortex, e.g. temporal lobe epilepsy. Contrast centrencephalic epilepsy (q.v.).
Focus	Limited area of disturbance, often delineated by phase reversal (q.v.).
Frequency	Number of complete cycles of a rhythm in one second.
Frequency analyser	Bank of filters each tuned to an individual frequency so that sections or epochs of the EEG, often 10 or 20 seconds, can be split into their components. A histogram is produced for each epoch, and these can readily be compared either between different sections of the same EEG or between EEGs done on different occasions.
Frequency spectrum	Range of frequencies composing the EEG, usually divided into the frequency bands delta, theta, alpha, beta.

Frontal intermittent rhythmic delta activity	Smooth, regular delta waves occurring in bursts over both frontal regions; abbreviation 'FIRDA'.
Gain	Ratio of output voltage to input voltage, i.e. the degree of amplification during the recording.
Gamma fast activity	Term no longer in use to describe 'fast' beta activity.
Generalised	Any form of cerebral activity seen widely over both hemispheres. Contrast localised or focal (q.v.).
Head cap	Slats generally of rubber or plastic tied under the chin which hold pad electrodes (q.v.) in place.
Hertz	Unit of frequency, either Hz/sec or c/sec (q.v.).
Hyperventilation	Form of activation routinely carried out during the EEG. The patient breathes deeply and regularly usually for three minutes. This causes a respiratory alkalosis which may enhance EEG abnormality (synonym 'over-breathing').
Hypsarrhythmia	Totally disorganised, very high voltage EEG containing irregular mixtures of spikes, sharp and slow waves. These discharges are usually more than 150 microvolts in amplitude and may exceed 500 microvolts; they may be multifocal, but generally the abnormality has a diffuse distribution. The record may show a type of 'burst-suppression' change during sleep, then periods of reduction in voltage of marked degree occur frequently. This

	EEG pattern is often associated with infantile spasms and mental subnormality.
Immaturity	Presence of features in the EEG characteristic of a younger age, e.g. posterior temporal slow waves, or poor regional differentiation of the alpha rhythm.
Inactive electrode	See 'White' lead.
Indifferent electrode	See 'White' lead.
In-phase signals	Signals such as 'mains hum' which affect the active and indifferent (or black and white) leads of the EEG amplifier in a similar fashion. They are discriminated against by the amplifier (see Common-mode rejection) allowing brain activity to be reproduced faithfully.
Input terminal 1	Internationally approved term for the time-hallowed 'black' lead (q.v.).
Input terminal 2	Internationally approved term for the time-hallowed 'white' lead (q.v.).
Intermittent	Term used to describe a wave or series of waves seen from time to time in the EEG (similar to Episode, Paroxysm, etc.)
Irregular	See Disorganised.
Irritative lesions	These lesions in contrast to most localised lesions lead to augmentation of background activities in a particular site rather than their diminution; they may occur, for example, with meningiomas.
Isoelectric	EEG in which there is no cerebral

activity. This implies 'brain death' (but see generally Chapter 13).

K complex	Combination of one or more high-voltage delta waves with spindles (Sigma rhythm). K complexes occur in a widespread fashion during stage 3 sleep, often as a result of an external stimulus.
Kappa rhythm	Term no longer in use to describe theta activity over the temporal lobes in relation to mentation.
Lambda waves	Sharply outlined positive triangular waves in the occipital region seen synchronously when the eyes are open and exploring an illuminated environment. Contrast lambdoid waves (q.v.).
Lambdoid waves	Triangular positive waves seen over the occipital poles synchronously in the second stage of sleep, with eyes shut (Contrast lambda waves, q.v.). They may have a more complex triphasic form and are generally of larger amplitude and longer duration. Lambdoid waves often occur in long runs lasting several seconds.
Lateralised	Involving one side of the head; compare Unilateral.
Lead	Term used to denote a single electrode and its attachment to the EEG machine.
Lesion	Term usually implying structural damage, contrasting with dysfunction (q.v.).
Local	EEG phenomenon which is seen to affect a channel or adjacent channels, often with phase reversal (q.v.).

Low-voltage EEG	Waking record characterised by activity of no more than 20 μ volts.
Mirror focus	Local spikes or sharp waves seen over homologous areas of cortex, e.g. temporal regions, with the implication that constant spiking in one area can cause, after many years, a similar change on the other side. This area then acts autonomously leading to spikes or sharp waves on its own account.
Mittens	Stereotyped complexes having a fast, followed by a slow, wave. These appear synchronously over the frontal regions usually in anaesthesia or drug-induced sleep.
Monophasic	Deflection either upwards or downwards, i.e. on one side of the base line; contrast diphasic and triphasic (q.v.).
Monopolar recording	Technique in which the potential from each electrode is compared with a relatively neutral source such as the ear lobe, a form of reference recording.
Montage	Combination of a number of derivations.
Morphology	The shape or form of EEG activity.
MSDA	Abbreviation for 'Monorhythmic Sinusoidal Delta Activity'. Synonyms include FIRDA (q.v.) or bifrontal delta activity. These terms imply dysfunction rather than structural abnormality (see also Projected abnormality).
Mu rhythm	Rhythm at 7 to 11 cycles per second in the rolandic regions usually persisting with the eyes open, often with a comb-like form and associated with an harmonically related beta rhythm. It is attenuated by real, imagined or

	intended movement, or tactile stimulation of a contralateral limb.
Naso-pharyngeal electrode	Rod electrode introduced through the nose and pressed against the naso-pharyngeal wall with its tip lying near the body of the sphenoid bone. An alternative method of recording to the sphenoidal leads (q.v.).
Noise	Any unwanted activity in the EEG, as distinct from the 'signal'. See Chapter 13 for details of means of enhancing 'signal' and reducing 'noise'.
Occipital rhythmic delta	Runs of fairly regular delta activity at 2½ – 3½ cycles per second occurring over the occipital region. Seen normally in young children especially just after eye closure. In older children it may imply posterior fossa disturbance.
Organisation	Degree to which physiological EEG rhythms conform to certain ideal characteristics displayed by a proportion of subjects in the same age group, free from personal or family history of neurological or psychiatric disorders or other conditions which may be associated with brain dysfunction. The organisation of physiological rhythms progresses from birth to adulthood and a poor degree of organisation may, but does not necessarily, imply abnormality.
Out of phase signals	Two waves with opposite phases.
Overbreathing	See Hyperventilation.
Pad electrode	Metal electrode, usually silver, covered

by cotton wool and lint and held in place by a head cap or harness.

Paper speed — Speed of movement of EEG paper usually expressed in centimetres per second. The most commonly used everyday paper speed in many countries is three centimetres per second.

Parietal humps — Stage-2 sleep phenomenon related to vertex sharp waves. Usually bilaterally symmetrical and synchronous.

Paradoxical (delta) response — Response in the form of generalised bisynchronous delta lasting several seconds following stimulation of comatose subject. Implies upper brain stem disturbance.

Paradoxical sleep — So called because the EEG resembles that of an alert subject and yet the person is difficult to rouse (synonym, 'REM sleep', q.v.).

Paroxysm — Phenomenon which appears and disappears abruptly and which is clearly distinguished from background activity by different amplitude, frequency and morphology. See also Epileptiform phenomena and Seizure discharge.

Pen — Term used to describe the write-out system which is most commonly ink on paper. In some EEG machines pens are replaced by ink jets, but the deflections are still in proportion to the change of potential in the channel. These 'jet' pens have much less inertia and other advantages over a straightforward pen system.

Period — Duration of a complete cycle of an individual EEG component.

Periodic	Term used to describe EEG waves or complexes which occur in sequence at an approximately regular rate. The intervals are generally of 1 to several seconds in duration (see Chapter 7).
Phase	Strictly, amplitude-time relations of sinusoidal waves, loosely time or polarity relations of different parts of a wave (or waves) as seen in a single trace, or of a wave (or waves) as recorded simultaneously in different channels.
Phase reversal	Phenomenon with two waves pointing together, created by the particular way that electrodes are connected in bipolar recording (see Chapter 3). This implies a localised electrical disturbance.
Photic stimulation	Technique of stroboscopic stimulation used during a routine EEG recording. In normals an occipital response results; but sometimes, in some forms of epilepsy for example, 'photosensitivity' (q.v.) occurs.
Photosensitivity	Widespread symmetrical repetitive discharge of spikes, sharp waves and slow waves resulting from stroboscopic stimulation, especially in some forms of idiopathic epilepsy. Seen in a minor form in a small percentage of normals. Also called the 'photo-paroxysmal response'.
PLEDS	Periodic lateralised epileptiform discharges, which occur in a variety of conditions (see Chapter 7). They usually have a repetition rate of more than one per second and are

associated with minor clinical epileptic phenomena in contrast to epilepsia partialis continuans.

Polarity convention — International agreement whereby EEG amplifiers are constructed so that a negative potential applied at the first input terminal or 'black' lead relative to the second input terminal or 'white' lead results in an upward deflection of the pen. A convention which does not necessarily apply in other biological fields.

Polygraphic recording — Recording of other physiological variables, e.g. ECG, respiration, etc., simultaneously with brain activity, on the same paper trace.

Polyphasic wave — Wave consisting of two or more components on alternate sides of the baseline; for example, a diphasic spike which has two components or a triphasic wave which has three components.

Posterior occipital spike-like waves of sleep — See Lambdoid waves.

Posterior temporal slow activity — Discrete, sharply contoured delta forms seen in the posterior temporal regions of young subjects. May persist into adult life, when they may be described as an 'immature' phenomenon.

Post-ictal EEG — Low amplitude recording characterised by relative absence of both 'epileptiform' and background activity. Reversion to previous EEG pattern may take up to 48 hours.

Projected abnormality	See MSDA, FIRDA, and Rhythm at a distance.
Projected patterns	Abnormal EEG activities, usually delta activity, resulting from disturbance at a site remote from the electrodes which are recording them. See MSDA, FIRDA, and Rhythm at a distance.
Provocative techniques	See Activation.
Quantity	Amount of activity in terms of amplitude and number of waves with respect to time.
Quiet sleep	Pattern of sleep seen in the neonate corresponding to slow-wave sleep in the adult.
Random	Recurring at inconstant time intervals.
Reactivity	Susceptibility of EEG rhythms to change following sensory stimulation; for example, eye opening attenuates the alpha rhythm.
Recording	Process of obtaining an EEG record, usually an ink-on-paper trace; synonym 'tracing'.
Reference electrode	A suitable reference electrode is selected to minimise the likelihood that it will pick up EEG activity. It is attached to the input terminal 2 or 'white' lead of the amplifier, whereas the active or exploring electrode is connected to the 1st input terminal or 'black' lead of the same amplifier. There are two main types of reference recording: the common reference or mono-polar and the common average reference recording (q.v.).

Reflex epilepsy	Epileptic attacks precipitated by specific stimuli, for example, photic stimulation. In rarer cases reading, music or other complex stimuli may lead to significant EEG and clinical phenomena.
Regional differentiation	The EEG in young children shows activity which is widely spread over the hemispheres, often most prominent in the Rolandic regions. With ageing this activity 'migrates' posteriorly so that there is a clear back-to-front differentiation in adults.
Regular	Term applying to waves or complexes of approximately constant period and relatively uniform appearance; for example, the alpha rhythm in the normal alert adult.
REM rebound	Increase in the amount of REM sleep above its normal 25% value, occurring after withdrawal from drugs, particularly barbiturates.
REM sleep	Rapid eye movement or paradoxical sleep; recurs periodically throughout the night. It is associated with a sudden change in the EEG from high-voltage irregular delta (slow-wave sleep) to a relatively low-voltage arhythmic record.
Rhythm	Activity of approximately constant period and morphology but not necessarily amplitude.
Rhythm at a distance	Usually episodic rhythmic delta activity occurring bilaterally in a particular site and implying dis-

turbance remote from that point; for example, frontal delta activity with a posterior fossa lesion (sometimes called 'projected' abnormality, q.v.).

Run	Colloquial term used for 'montage' (q.v.).
Scalp electrode	Electrode held against, attached to or inserted into the scalp, depending on whether pad, stick-on or needle electrodes are used.
Seizure discharge	Disturbance which 'builds up' and 'dies down', usually rhythmic with changing frequency and amplitude during its course. These discharges are commonly localised in one area, but several areas may be affected at different times, for instance in an infant. The duration of these discharges may be variable, from about a second to several minutes, with longer discharges spreading to homologous areas on the opposite side. Similar discharges may be seen with or without a definite clinical concomitant. In this latter instance they are called 'subclinical'.
Sensitivity	Ratio of input voltage to output pen deflection in an EEG channel measured in microvolts per millimetre; contrast Gain (q.v.).
Sharp and slow wave complex	Sequence of a sharp, followed by a slow wave. One of the so called 'epileptiform' patterns.
Sharp wave	Transient phenomenon clearly distinguished from the background activity. It has a pointed outline at

	conventional paper speeds and has a duration of 70 to 200 milliseconds; that is, it lasts 1/14 to 1/5 seconds approximately (compare spike).
Sigma rhythm	Episodic phenomenon comprising spindle-like bursts of rhythmic activity at 10 to 14 cycles per second, of 1 to 2 seconds duration. These are usually of 20 to 50 microvolts and occur in equal amounts, but not necessarily simultaneously, in the fronto-parietal regions. In children the spindles often appear at quite different times on the two sides, whereas they are much more often seen simultaneously or synchronously in adults.
Signal	Term used to describe the activity which the electroencephalographer wishes to examine; for example, the cortical evoked response. It is time-locked to a stimulus while the on-going background activity is not and can be regarded as 'noise' (see Chapter 13).
Silence, record of electro-cerebral	EEG which contains no cerebral activity as in 'brain death'. See Isoelectric recording.
Sinusoidal	In ordinary EEG work implies waves with a smooth outline and regular form; strictly, artificially generated waves whose upwards deflection from and return to the baseline is followed by an identical deflection downwards.
Sleep recording	May be relatively brief, e.g. ½–¾ hours, with an attempt to activate 'epileptic' discharges; or 'all night' to find, for example, changes in pro-

portion of REM and other types of sleep. There are many phenomena seen in sleep, e.g. vertex sharp waves, K complexes, some of which can be confused with abnormal wave forms.

Sleep spindles — Bursts of activity at 12 to 14 cycles per second which are often diffuse but higher over the frontal regions, seen during stage 2 sleep (synonym, 'sigma rhythm').

Sleep stages — Distinctive phases of sleep demonstrated on EEG with polygraphic recordings of other variables; for example, eye movements and activity in voluntary muscles.

Sleep staging — Applies particularly to overnight sleep recordings. These are usually rated by eye, each page or section being given a number depending on the stage of sleep that it shows, according to an international manual (see Chapter 10).

Slow wave — Waves of duration longer than alpha waves, that is over 1/8th of a second; can be either theta or delta activity (q.v.).

Sphenoidal electrode — Needle or wire electrode inserted through the soft tissue of the face below the zygomatic arch with the tip lying near the base of the skull in the region of the foramen ovale, thus recording from the inferior and medial aspects of the temporal lobe.

Sphenoidal recording — EEG in which sphenoidal leads (q.v.) are used usually combined with the administration of intravenous barbiturate or other agents; for example, bemegride.

Spike	Defined as a wave clearly distinguished from the background activity with a duration of 1/12th of a second or less (80 msec) (compare Sharp wave).
Spike and wave activity	Complexes of one spike followed by a wave which appear in all regions at once and recur at the rate of 3 per second. These are typical of petit mal. Atypical spike and wave, for example with a different repetition rate, may be localised or generalised and occur in a wide variety of conditions associated with epilepsy (see Chapter 4).
Spikes, 14 and 6 per second positive	Runs of positive spikes at 14 and 6 per second seen over the temporal regions with monopolar recording (either linked ear or opposite ear reference) principally in young adults during light sleep. Their significance is hotly disputed.
Spindled activity	Activity which waxes and wanes, especially alpha, with no particular clinical significance.
Stereotactic depth electro-encephalogram	Recording of the electrical activity of the brain by means of electrodes implanted in the brain surface using stereotactic means.
Stick-on electrodes	Disc electrodes attached to the scalp with either collodion or other types of adhesive.
Stroboscope	Apparatus which produces very brief bright flashes of light, used during photic stimulation. The rate of the flash can be controlled by the turn of a knob.

Structural lesion	Term taken to imply a destructive process in a particular site; for example, tumour, haemorrhage, or abscess. In contrast to a dysfunctional process (q.v.).
Sub-clinical seizure discharge	See Seizure discharge.
Subdural electrode	Electrode inserted under the dural covering of the brain which may be left in place for recording for hours or days.
Superimposition	Technique for delineating cortical-evoked responses from the background activity. It involves the display of each individual response successively on a cathode ray oscilloscope and photographing it on a single photographic plate. Largely superseded by 'averaging' (q.v.).
Suppression	Term used to describe occasions in the EEG when cerebral activity suddenly diminishes in voltage or disappears completely, as in the burst-suppression pattern (q.v.). It is observed in deep anaesthesia or, for example, following cerebral anoxic episodes.
Synchronisation	Implies that the activity occurs at exactly the same time on the two sides of the head; for example, normal alpha waves. It suggests a mid-line origin or pacemaker for the activity (see Chapter 2).
Ten-twenty system	System of standardised scalp electrode placement agreed internationally. The placement is determined by measurement of the head from external bony landmarks taking 10% or 20%

	segments of, for example, the circumference of the skull.
Theta	Used to indicate waves or a rhythm with a frequency of from 4 to 7½ cycles per second which occur in the resting record. Each wave will have a period of 1/4 to 1/8 of a second.
Time constant	Name applied to the low frequency filtering of the EEG channel. In fact it depends on the resistive and capacitative characteristics of the channel (see Cooper *et al.* (1974) for technical details).
Tracé alternant	A discontinuous EEG pattern observed in the neonate. It may be normal depending on the state of the patient, the exact phemomena seen, and the gestational age.
Transient	Any single wave (spike, sharp wave, etc.) or brief complex standing out from the background.
Triphasic waves	Delta waves with a specific configuration, an up-going phase followed by a sharpened down-going phase, and an up-going third phase before returning to the baseline (see Chapter 7). Usually these waves are seen synchronously, and with a frontal emphasis. They are characteristic of hepatic encephalopathy.
Unilateral	Occurring only on one side.
Unipolar	Synonym for 'monopolar,' one form of referential EEG recording (q.v.).
Vertex sharp waves	Paroxysmal phenomenon of stage-2 sleep occurring on a low-voltage fast background. Seen synchronously and

usually symmetrically with a phase reversal at the vertex. They merge into the phenomenon called 'biparietal humps', a term no longer in general use.

Wave	Any transient change of potential difference in the EEG.
'White lead'	Second or indifference input to a biological amplifier. Because of the EEG convention a negative potential, for example, at the white lead causes a downward deflection of the pen, and vice versa.

Bibliography

General

Brazier M.A.B. (1968) *The Electrical Activity of the Nervous System.* Pitman Medical, London.

Cooper, R., Osselton, J.W. and Shaw, J.C., (2nd ed. 1974) *EEG Technology,* Butterworth, London.

Craib, A.R., and Most, M., (1973) *The EEG Handbook,* ed. Low, M.D., Beckman Instruments, New York.

Gibbs, F.A. and Gibbs, E.L. (1941) *Atlas of Electro-encephalography,* Cambridge, Mass.

Gibbs, F.A. and Gibbs, E.L. (1951) (1952) (1964) *Atlas of Electroencephalography,* Cambridge, Mass.

Gloor, P. (1969) 'Hans Berger on the electroencephalogram of man,' *Electroencephalography and Clinical Neuro-physiology,* Supplement 28.

Hill, D. and Parr, G. (1963) *Electroencephalography,* Macdonald, London.

Kellaway, P. and Petersen, I. (1968) *Neurological and Electroencephalographic correlate of studies in infancy.* Grune and Stratton, New York and London.

Kiloh, L.G., McComas, A.J. and Osselton, J.W. (1972) *Clinical Electroencephalography,* Butterworth, London.

Kooi, K.A. (1971) *Fundamentals of electroencephalography,* Harper & Row, New York and London.

Laidlaw, J. and Stanton, J.B. (1966) *The EEG in Clinical Practice,* Livingstone, London.

Margerison, J.H., St. John-Loe, P. and Binnie, C.D. (1967) 'Electroencephalography,' in *Manual of Psychophysio-logical Methods,* ed. Venables, P.H. and Martin, I., North Holland, Amsterdam.

Oswald, I., (1962) *Sleeping and Waking,* Elsevier, Amsterdam.

Walter, Grey (1951, 1963) *The Living Brain,* Duckworth, London.

Chapter 1

Jasper, H.H. (1958) 'Report of the committee of methods of clinical examination in electroencephalography,' *Electroencephalography and Clinical Neurophysiology, 10,* 370.

Matthews, W.B. (1973) 'The clinical value of routine electroencephalography,' *Journal of Royal College of Physicians of London, 7,* 207.

Pappworth, M. (1974) 'Neurologists need their heads examined,' *Mims Magazine,* London.

Chapter 2

Adrian, E.D. and Matthews, B.H.C. (1934a) 'Interpretation of potential waves in the cortex,' *Journal of Physiology, 81,* 440.

Adrian, E.D. and Matthews, B.H.C. (1934b) 'Berger rhythms: Potential changes from the occipital lobes in man,' *Brain, 57,* 355.

Andersen, P. and Andersson, S.A. (1968) *Physiological Basis of the Alpha Rhythm,* Appleton-Century-Croft, New York, 235.

Bremer, F. (1935) 'Cerveau isolé et physiologie du sommeil,' *Comptes rendus des séances de la Société Biologique, 118,* 1235.

Cabral, R. and Scott, D.F. (1975), in press. 'The degree of alpha asymmetry and its relation to handedness in neuropsychiatric referrals,' *Acta Neurologica Scandinavica.*

Da Silver Lopes, F.H., Van Lierops, T.H.M.T., Schrifer, C.F. and Storm Van Leeuren, W., 'Organisation of thalamic and cortical alpha rhythms, spectra and coherences,' *Electroencephalography and Clinical Neurophysiology,* 1973, *35,* 627.

Editorial (1974) 'Computer-assisted tomography of the brain,' *Lancet, 2,* 1052.

Ellul, R. (1972) 'The genesis of the EEG,' in *International review of Neurobiology,* ed. Pfeiffer, C.C. and Smythes, C.C. Academic Press, London.

Harding, G.F.A. (1971) 'The use of automated low frequency wave analysis in quantitive electroencephalography,' in Stocker, G., *Assessment in Cerebrovascular Insufficiency,* Thieme, Stuttgart.

Lindsley, D.B., Schreiner, L.H., Knowles, W.B. and Magoun, H.W. (1950) 'Behavioural and EEG changes following chronic brain stem lesions in cats,' *Electroencephalography and Clinical Neurophysiology, 2,* 483.

Lippold, O.C. (1973) *The Origin of the Alpha Rhythm,* Heinemann Medical, London.

Margerison, J.H., Anderson, W. and Dawson, M. C. (1964) 'Plasma sodium and EEG during the menstrual cycle of normal human females,' *Electroencephalography and Clinical Neurophysiology, 17,* 540.

Scott, D. and Bickford, R.G. (1969) 'Stimulus indicators of human lambda responses,' *Archives of Neurology, 21,* 277.

Scott, D.F., Schwartz, M.S., Farrant, G.W. and Speirs, C.F. (1974) 'The importance of methodology in drug studies using EEG,' *Electroencephalography and Clinical Neurophysiology, 37,* 670.

Chapter 3

Decker, D.A. Jr. and Knott, J.R. (1972) 'The EEG in instrinsic supratentorial brain tumours: a comparative evaluation,' *Electroencephalography and Clinical Neurophysiology, 33,* 303.

Fischer-Williams, M., Last, S.L., Lyberi, G. and Northfield, D.W.C. (1962) 'Clinico-EEG study of 128 gliomas and 50 intracranial metastatic tumours,' *Brain, 85,* 1.

Magnus, O., Storm van Leeuwen, W. and Cobb, W.A. (eds) (1961). 'Electroencephalography and cerebral tumours,' *Electroencephalography and Clinical Neurophysiology,* Supplement 19, Elsevier, Amsterdam.

Prior, P.F.P. (1968) 'Electroencephalographic studies in patients after removal of intracranial menginiomas,' *Acta Neurologica Scandinavica, 44,* 107.

Rowan, A.J., Rudolf, N. de M. and Scott, D.F. (1974) 'EEG prediction of brain metastases,' *Journal of Neurology, Neurosurgery and Psychiatry, 37,* 888.

Silverman, D. and Groff, R.A. (1957) 'Brain tumour depth determination by electroencephalographic recordings during sleep,' *Archives of Neurology and Psychiatry, 78,* 15.

Strang, R., and Ajmone Marsan, C. (1961) 'Brain metastases,' *Archives of Neurology, 4,* 20.

Van der Drift, J.H.A. (1957) *The Significance of Electroencephalography for the Diagnosis and Localisation of Cerebral tumours,* Stenfert Kroeses, Leiden.

Walter, W.G. (1936), 'The location of cerebral tumours by electroencephalography,' *Lancet, 2,* 305.

Chapter 4

Ames, F. (1974) 'Cinefilm and EEG recording during hand waving attacks of an epileptic photo-sensitive child,' *Electroencephalography and Clinical Neurophysiology, 37,* 301.

Binnie, C.D., Darby, C.E. and Hindley, A.T. (1973) 'Electroencephalographic changes in epileptics while viewing television,' *British Medical Journal, 4,* 378.

Brazier, M.A.B. (1973) ed. *Epilepsy: Its Phenomena in Man,* UCLA Forum in Medical Sciences No. 17, Academic Press, New York and London.

Critchley, M.A. and Scott, D.F. (1975) 'Musicogenic Epilepsy,' in *Music and Brain,* Heinemann Medical, London.

Currie S., Heathfield, K.W.G., Henson, R.A. and Scott, D.F. (1971) 'Clinical course and prognosis of temporal lobe epilepsy,' *Brain, 94,* 173.

Hutt, S.J., Lee, D. and Ounsted, C. (1972) 'Digit memory and evoked discharges in four light-sensitive epileptic children,' *Developmental Medicine and Child Neurology, 5,* 559.

Jeavons, P.M. and Harding, G.F.A. (1970) 'Television epilepsy,' *Lancet, 1,* 926.

Jeavons, P.M., Harding, G.F.A. and Panayiotopoulos, C.P. (1971) 'Photosensitive epilepsy and driving,' *Lancet, 1,* 1125.

Legg, N.J., Gupta, P.C. and Scott, D.F. (1973) 'Epilepsy following cerebral abscess: a clinical study of 70 patients,' *Brain, 96,* 259.

Lennox-Buchthal, M.A. (1973) 'Febrile convulsions – a reappraisal,' *Electroencephalography and Clinical Neurophysiology,* Supplement 32.

Margerison, J.H. and Corsellis, J.A.N. (1966) 'Epilepsy and the temporal lobes,' *Brain, 89,* 499.

Morgan, H.M. and Scott, D.F. (1970) 'EEG activation in epilepsies other than petit mal,' *Epilepsia, 11,* 255.

Pampiglione, G. and Kerridge, J. (1956) 'EEG abnormalities from the temporal lobe studied with sphenoidal electrodes,' *Journal of Neurology, Neurosurgery and Psychiatry, 19,* 117.

Penfield, W. (1969) 'Epilepsy, neurophysiology and some brain mechanisms related to consciousness,' in *Basic Mechanisms of the Epilepsies,* ed. Jasper, H.H. Ward, A.A. and Pope, A., Churchill, London.

Penry, K.J. (1973) *'Behavioural Correlates of Generalised Spike-Wave Discharge in the electroencephalogram,* Academic Press, New York, 171–88.

Prensky, L., DeVivo, C. and Palkes, H. (1971) 'Severe bradykinesia as a manifestation of toxicity to antiepileptic medications,' *Journal of Pediatrics, 700,* 704.

Rowan, A.J. and Scott, D.F. (1970) 'Major status epilepticus,' *Acta Neurologica Scandinavica, 46,* 573.

Schwartz, M.S. and Scott, D.F. (1971) 'Isolated petit-mal status presenting de novo in middle age,' *Lancet, 2,* 1399.

Scott, D.F. (1973) *About Epilepsy,* Duckworth, London.

Wilson, P.J.E. (1973) 'The surgical treatment of epilepsy,' *British Journal of Hospital Medicine, 11,* 161.

Zivin, L. and Ajmone Marsan, C. (1968) 'Incidence and prognostic significance of epileptiform activity in the EEG of non-epileptic subjects,' *Brain, 91,* 751,

Chapter 5

Croft, P.B., Heathfield, K.W.G. and Swash, M. (1973) 'Differential diagnosis of transient amnesia,' *British Medical Journal, 4,* 593.

Ellington, A., Arranibar, A. and Torres, F. (1970) 'Evaluation of cerebrovascular disease,' *Archives of Neurology, 23,* 404.

Editorial (1974) 'Computer-assisted tomography of the brain,' *Lancet, 2,* 1052.

Fenton, G. (1974) 'The straightforward EEG in psychiatric practice,' *Proceedings of the Royal Society of Medicine, 67,* 911.

Hanington, E. (1967) 'A preliminary report on tyramine headache,' *British Medical Journal, 2,* 550.

Lundervold, A. Harige, E. and Loken, A.Z. (1956) 'Unusual EEG in unconscious patient with brain stem atrophy,' *Electroencephalography and Clinical Neurophysiology, 8,* 665.

Margerison, J.H., Binnie, C.D., and McCaul, I.R. (1970) 'Electroencephalographic signs employed in the location of ruptured intracranial arterial aneurysms,' *Electroencephalography and Clinical Neurophysiology 28,* 296.

Moffett, A., Swash, M. and Scott, D.F. (1972) 'Effect of tyramine in migraine: a double blind study,' *Journal of Neurology, Neurosurgery and Psychiatry, 35,* 496.

Moffett, A.M. Swash, M. and Scott, D.F. (1974) 'The effect of chocolate in migraine: a double blind study,' *Journal of Neurology, Neurosurgery and Psychiatry, 37,* 445.

Scott, D.F., Moffett, A. and Swash M. (1972) 'Observations on the relationship of migraine and epilepsy,' *Epilepsia, 13,* 365.

Van der Drift, J.H. and Magnus, O. (1961) 'The EEG in cerebral ischaemic lesions: Correlations with clinical and pathological findings,' *Cerebral Anoxia and the Electroencephalogram,* ed. Gastaut, H. and Meyers, J.S., Thomas Springfield, Ill.

Chapter 6

Bickford, R.G., and Klass, Donald W. (1966) 'EEG changes with acute and chronic head injury,' *Head Injury Conference Proceedings,* ed. Caveness, W.F. and Earl Walker, A. Lippincott, Philadelphia.

Courjan, J.A. (1969) 'Post-traumatic epilepsy in electro-clinical practice,' in *Late Effects of Head Injury,* Walker, A.E., Caveness, W.F. and Critchley, M. Thomas, Springfield, Ill.

Dow, R.S., Ulett, C. and Reaf. J. (1944) 'Electroencephalographic studies immediately following head injury,' *American Journal of Psychiatry, 101,* 174.

Jennett, B. (1972) 'Prognosis after severe head injury,' *Clinical Neurosurgery, 19,* 200.

Jennett, B. (1974). 'Early traumatic epilepsy,' *Archives of Neurology, 30,* 395.

Jennett B., Plum, F. (1972) 'Persistent vegetative state after brain damage, *Lancet, 1,* 734.

Jennett, B. Teather, D. and Bennies, B. (1973) 'Epilepsy after head injury,' *Lancet 2,* 652.

Pampus, F. and Grote, W. (1956) 'Elektrenkephalographie und klinische Befunde bei Arch. Psychiat. Boxern und ihre Bedeutung für die Pathophysiologie der traumatischen Hirnshadigung,' *Archiv für Psychiatrie und Nervenkrankheiten, 194,* 152.

Prior, P.F. (1973) *The EEG in Acute Cerebral Anoxia,* Excerpta Medica, Amsterdam.

Rapport, R.L. and Penry, J.K. (1972) 'Pharmacological prophylaxis of post-traumatic epilepsy,' *Epilepsia, 13,* 295.

Teasdale, G. and Jennett, B. (1974) 'Assessment of coma and impairment of consciousness,' *Lancet, 1,* 81.

Chapter 7.

Bayliss, S.G., Jenkins, A.M. and Rickell, M. (1971), 'Subacute sclerosing panencephalitis,' *Proceedings of the Electrophysiological Technicians' Asociation, 18,* 163.

Bickford, R.G., and Butt, H.R. (1955) 'Hepatic coma: the electroencephalographic pattern,' *Journal of Clinical Investigations, 34,* 790.

Burger, L.J., Rowan, A.J. and Goldensohn, E.S. (1972) 'Creutzfeld Jakob Disease: an electroencephalographic study,' *Archives of Neurology, 26,* 428.

Chatrian, G.E., Shaw, C.M. and Leffman, H. (1964) 'The significance of periodic lateralized epileptiform discharges in EEG: an electrographic, clinical and pathological study,' *Electroencephalography and Clinical Neurophysiology, 17,* 177.

Editorial, (1972) 'Herpes encephalitis,' *British Medical Journal, 1,* 582.

Engel, G.L. and Romano, J. (1959) 'Delirium, a syndrome of cerebral insufficiency,' *Journal of Chronic Diseases, 9,* 260.

Ibrahim, M.M. and Jeavons, P.M. (1974) 'The value of electroencephalography in the diagnosis of subacute sclerosing panencephalitis,' *Developmental Medicine and Child Neurology, 16,* 295.

Illis, L.S. and Taylor, F.M. (1972) 'The electroencephalogram in herpes simplex encephalitis,' *Lancet, 1,* 718.

Jooma, O.V., Pennybacker, J.B. and Tutton, G.K. (1951) 'Brain abscess: aspiration, drainage or excision?', *Journal of Neurology, Neurosurgery and Psychiatry 14,* 308.

Nevin, S., McMenemey, W.H., Behrman, S. and Jones, D.P. (1960) 'Subacute spongiform encephalopathy: a subacute form of encephalopathy attributable to vascular dysfunction (spongiform cerebral atrophy),' *Brain 83,* 519.

Pampiglione, G. (1964) 'Prodromal phase of measles. Some neurophysiological studies,' *British Medical Journal, 2,* 1296.

Schwartz, M.S., Prior, P.F. and Scott, D.F. (1973) 'The occurrence and evolution in the EEG of a lateralized periodic phenomenon,' *Brain, 96,* 613.

Swash, M. and Rowan, A.J. (1972) 'Electroencephalographic criteria of hypocalcaemia and hypercalcaemia,' *Archives of Neurology, 26,* 218.

Upton, A. and Gumpert, J. (1970) 'Electroencephalography in diagnosis of herpes-simplex encephalitis,' *Lancet, 1,* 650.

Chapter 8.

Aird, R.B. and Cohen, P. (1950) 'Electroencephalography in cerebral palsy,' *Journal of Paediatrics, 37,* 448.

Baldock, G.R. and Walter, W.G. (1946) 'A new electronic analyser,' *Electronic Engineering, 18,* 339.

Bowers, B.D. (1974) 'Fits, faints and "funny turns" in young children,' *British Journal of Hospital Medicine, 12,* 527.

Churchill, J.A. and Rodin, E.A. (1968) 'Asymmetry of alpha activity in children,' *Developmental Medicine and Child Neurology, 10,* 77.

Corbin, H.P.F. and Bickford, R.G. (1955) 'Studies of the electroencephalogram of normal children: comparison of visual and automatic frequency analyses,' *Electroencephalography and Clinical Neurophysiology, 7,* 15.

Falconer, M.A. (1974) 'Mesial temporal (Ammon's horn) sclerosis as a common cause of epilepsy, aetiology, treatment and prevention,' *Lancet, 2,* 767.

Forfar, J.O. (1974) 'Biochemical fits in the newborn,' *Proceedings of Royal Society of Medicine, 67,* 375.

Gregoriades, A. and Pampiglione, G. (1966) 'Seizures in children with Down's Syndrome (Mongolism),' *Electroencephalography and Clinical Neurophysiology, 21,* 307.

Harris, R. and Tizard, J.P.M. (1960) 'The electroencephalogram in neonatal convulsions,' *Journal of Pediatrics, 51,* 501.

Jeavons, P. (1974) 'Infantile spasms,' in *Handbook of Clinical Neurology,* vol. 15, North Holland, Amsterdam.

Pampiglione, G. (1973) 'The effect of metabolic disorders on brain activity,' *Journal of the Royal College of Physicians of London, 1,* 347.

Parmelee, H., Akayama, Y., Schultz M.A., Wenner, W.H., Schulte, F.J. and Stern, B., (1968) 'The electroencephalogram in active and quiet sleep in infants,' in *Clinical Electroencephalography of Children,* ed. Kellaway, P. and Petersen, I., Almqvist & Wiksell, Stockholm.

Prechtl, H.F.R., Akayama, Y., Zimkim, P. and Grant, D.K. (1968) 'Polygraphic studies of the full term newborn in studies in infancy,' in *Clinical and Developmental Medicine No. 27,* ed, Keith, R. and Box, M., Spastics International Medical Publications in association with Heinemann Medical, London.

Smith, S.M. and Honigsberger, L. (1973) 'EEG and personality factors in baby batterers,' *British Medical Journal, 3,* 20.

Wilson, P.J.E. (1970) 'Infantile hemiplegia', *Brain 93,* 147.

Chapter 9

Betts, T.A., Kalra, P.L., Cooper, R. and Jeavons, P.M. (1968) 'Epileptic fits as a probable side-effect of amitriptyline,' *Lancet, 1,* 390.

Dallos, V. and Heathfield, K.W. (1969) 'Iatrogenic epilepsy due to anti-depressant drugs,' *British Medical Journal, 4,* 80.

Fenton, G.W. (1974) 'The straightforward EEG in psychiatric practice,' *Proceedings of the Royal Society of Medicine, 67,* 911.

Fenton, G.W., and Scotton, L. (1967) 'Personality and the alpha rhythm,' *British Journal of Psychiatry, 113,* 122.

Fenton, G.W., Tennent, T.G., Comish, K.A. and Rattrey, N (1971) 'EEG and sex chromosome abnormalities,' *British Journal of Psychiatry, 119,* 185.

Fenwick, C., Fenton, G.W., Dollimore, J., Rutter, M., and Yule, W. (1975) 'Intelligence and power spectra in adolescent boys,' *Electroencephalography and Clinical Neurophysiology, 38,* 210.

Flor-Henry, P. (1969) 'Psychosis and temporal lobe epilepsy,' *Epilepsia, 10,* 363.

Gjessing, L.R., Harding, G.F.A., Jenner, F.A. and Johannessen, N.B. (1967) 'The EEG in three cases of periodic catatonia,' *British Journal of Psychiatry, 113,* 1271.

Harding, G.F.A. (1974) 'The EEG in affective disorders,' in *Handbook of Clinical Neurophysiology,* Elsevier, Amsterdam.

Hopkins, A. (1973) 'Pretending to be unconscious,' *Lancet, 2,* 312.

Letemendia, F. and Pampiglione, G. (1958) 'Clinical and electroencephalographic observation in Alzheimer's disease,' *Journal of Neurology, Neurosurgery and Psychiatry, 21,* 167.

Scott, D.F., Heathfield, K.W.G., Toone, B., and Margerison, J.H. (1972) 'The EEG in Huntington's Chorea: a clinical and neuropathological study,' *Journal of Neurology, Neurosurgery and Psychiatry, 35,* 97.

Scott, D.F. and Schwartz, M.S. (1975) 'The EEG in schizophrenic and depressive states,' *British Journal of Psychiatry, 126,* 408.

Sishta, S.K., Troupe, A., Marszalek, K.S. and Kremer, N.M. (1974) 'Huntington's Chorea: an electroencephalographic and psychometric study,' *Electroencephalography and Clinical Neurophsiology, 36,* 387.

Slater, E., Beard, A.W. and Glithero, E. (1963) 'The schizophrenia-like psychoses of epilepsy,' *British Journal of Psychiatry, 109,* 95.

Taylor, D.C. (1972) 'Mental state and temporal lobe epilepsy,' *Epilepsia, 13,* 727.

Volavka, J., Feldstein, S., Abrams, R., Dornbush, R. and Fink, M. (1972) 'EEG and clinical change after bilateral and unilateral electroconvulsive therapy,' *Electroencephalography and Clinical Neurophysiology, 32,* 631.

Walter, G., Cooper, R., Aldridge, V.J., McCallum, W.C., and Winter, A.L. (1964) 'Contingent Negative Variation: an electric sign of sensori-motor association and expectancy in the human brain,' *Nature, 203,* 380.

Chapter 10

Aserinsky, E. and Kleitman, N. (1955) 'Two types of ocular motility occurring during sleep,' *Journal of Applied Physiology, 8,* 1.

Brezinova, V. and Oswald, I. (1972) 'Sleep after a bedtime beverage,' *British Medical Journal, 2,* 431.

Fischer, C., Kahn, E., Edwards, A., Davis, D.M. and Fine J. (1974) 'A psycho-physiological study of nightmares and night terrors,' *Journal of Nervous and Mental Disease, 158,* 174.

Gross, M.M., Goodenough, D., Tobin, N., Highpart, E., Lepore, D., Perstein, A., Sorrote, M., Debeanco, J., Fuller, R. and Khrishner, I. (1966) 'Sleep disturbance and hallucinations in the acute alcoholic psychosis,' *Journal of Mental and Nervous Diseases, 142,* 493.

Haider, I. and Oswald, I. (1970) 'Late brain recovery processes after drug overdose,' *Electroencephalography and Clinical Neurophysiology, 29,* 326.

Johns, M.W., Large, A.A., Masterton, J.P. and Dudley, H.A.F. (1974) 'Sleep and delirium after open heart surgery,' *British Journal of Surgery, 61,* 377.

Malpas, A., Rowan, A.J., Joyce, C.R.B. and Scott, D.F., (1970) 'Persistent behavioural and electroencephalographic changes after single doses of nitrazepam and amylobarbitone sodium,' *British Medical Journal, 2,* 762.

Malpas, A., Legg, N.J. and Scott, D.F. (1974) 'Effects of hypnotics on anxious patients,' *British Journal of Psychiatry, 124,* 482.

Oswald, I. and Priest, R.G. (1965) 'Five weeks to escape the sleeping pill habit,' *British Medical Journal, 2,* 1093.

Parkes, J.D., Marsden, C.D. (1974) 'Narcolepsy,' *British Journal of Hospital Medicine, 12,* 325.

Rechtschaffen, A. and Kales, A. (eds) (1968) *A Manual of Standardised Technology, Techniques, and Scoring System for Sleep Stages in Human Subjects,* U.S. Government printing offices, Washington D.C.

Speirs, C.F., Virden, S. and Scott, D.F. (1972) 'A simultaneous plasma level and EEG assessment of an oral hypnotic ethinamate,' *European Journal of Pharmacology, 20,* 127.

Chapter 11

Binnie, C.D., Prior, P.F., Lloyd, D.S.L., Scott, D.F. and Margerison, J.H. (1970) 'Electroencephalographic prediction of fatal anoxic brain damage after resuscitation from cardiac arrest,' *British Medical Journal, 4,* 265.

Brierly, J.B., Adams, J.H., Fraham, D.I. and Simpson, J.A. (1971) 'Neocortical death after cardiac arrest,' *Lancet, 1,* 560.

Maynard, D., Prior, P.F. and Scott, D.F., (1969) 'Device for continuous monitoring of cerebral activity in resuscitated patients,' *British Medical Journal, 4,* 545.

Maynard, D. and Prior, P.F. (1973) 'A predictive instrument to assist with interpretation of EEGs of patients resuscitated after cardiac arrest,' *Electroencephalography and Clinical Neurophysiology, 35,* 744.

Pampiglione, G. and Harden, A. (1968) 'Resuscitation after cardiocirculatory arrest,' *Lancet, 1,* 1261.

Prior, P.F., Maynard, D.E., Sheaff, P.S., Simpson, B.R., Strunin, L., Weaver, E.J.M. and Scott, D.F. (1971)

'Monitoring cerebral function: clinical experience with new device for continuous recording of electrical activity of brain,' *British Medical Journal, 2,* 736.

Prior, P.F. (1973) *The EEG in Acute Cerebral Anoxia,* Excerpta Medica, Amsterdam.

Prior, P.F., Scott, D.F. and Maynard, D.E. (1974) 'The EEG in assessment of brain death,' *Proceedings from First International Intensive Care Congress,* London.

Silverman, D., Saunders, M.G., Schwab, R.S. and Masland, R.L. (1969) 'Cerebral death and the electroencephalogram: Report of the Ad Hoc Committee of the American Electroencephalographic Society on EEG criteria for determination of cerebral death,' *Journal of the American Medical Association, 209,* 1505.

Skillman, J.J. (1974) 'Ethical dilemmas in the care of the critically ill,' *Lancet, 2,* 634.

Chapter 12

Coursen, G., Domino, E.F. and Breer, R.L. (1969) 'Electroencephalographic effects of ketamine anaesthesia in children,' *Anaesthesia and Analgesia: Current researches, 48,* 141.

Faulconer, A. and Bickford, R.G. (1960) *Servo Anaesthesia in Electroencephalography in Anaesthesiology,* Thomas, Springfield, Ill.

Magoun, H.W. (1963) *The Waking Brain,* Thomas, Springfield, Ill.

Ramsay, M.A.E., Savage, T.M., Simpson, B.R.J. and Goodwin, R. (1974) 'Controlled sedation with alphaxalone-alphadolone,' *British Medical Journal, 2,* 656.

Sadove, M.J., Becker, K.A.D. and Gibbs, F.A. (1967) *Electroencephalography for Anaesthesiologists and Surgeons,* Lippincott, Philadelphia and Pitman Medical, London.

Schwartz, M.S., Colvin, M.P., Prior, P.F. Strunin, L., Simpson, B.R., Weaver, E.J.M. and Scott, D.F. (1973) 'The Cerebral Function Monitor: its value in predicting the neurological outcome in patients undergoing cardiopulmonary by-pass,' *Anaesthesia, 28,* 611.

Schwartz, M.S., Virden, S. and Scott, D.F. (1974) 'Effects of ketamine on the electroencephalograph,' *Anaesthesia, 29,* 135.

Scott, D.F. and Virden, S., (1972) 'Comparison of the effect of Althesin with other induction agents on electroencephalographic patterns,' *Postgraduate Medical Journal* (June Supplement), 93.

Chapter 13

Cody, D.T.R., Klass, D.W. and Bickford, R.G., (1967) 'Cortical audiometry: an objective measure of evaluating auditory acuity in an awake and sleeping man,' *Transactions of the American Academy of Ophalmology and Otorhinolaryngology, 71,* 81.

Dawson, G.D. (1947) 'Cerebral responses to electrical stimulation of peripheral nerve in man,' *Journal of Neurology, Neurosurgery and Psychiatry, 10,* 134.

Halliday, A.M., McDonald, W.I. and Mushin, J. (1972) 'Delayed visual evoked responses in optic neuritis,' *Lancet, 1,* 982.

Kornhuber, H.H. and Deecke, L. (1965) 'Hirnpotentialänderungen bei Wilkürbewegungen und passiven Bewegungen des Menschen: Bereitschaftspotential und reafferente Potentiale,' *Pflugers Archiv für die gesamte Physiologie des Menschen und der Tiere, 284,* 1.

Lehtinen, L.O.J. and Bergström, L. (1970) 'Naso-ethnoidal electrode for recording the electrical activity of the inferior surface of the frontal lobe,' *Electroencephalography and Clinical Neurophysiology, 29,* 303.

McCallum, W.C. and Knott, G.R. (1973) 'Event-related slow potentials of the brain: their relations to behaviour,' *Electroencephalography and Clinical Neurophysiology* Supplement 33.

Regan, D., (1972) *Evoked Potentials in Psychology, Sensory Physiology and Clinical Medicine,* Chapman & Hall, London.

Solomon, G. and Elberling, C. (1971) 'Cochlear nerve potentials recorded from the ear in man,' *Otolaryngology, 71.* 319.

Scott, D.F. and Bickford, R.G., (1969) 'Stimulus indicators of summated human lambda response,' *Archives of Neurology, 21,* 277.

Scott, D.F., Hoffman, H.J. and Bickford, R.G., (1969) 'Evoked potentials (Lambda waves) relating to the non-additive properties of the visual sensory in-flow,' *Perceptual and Motor Skills, 29,* 307.

Small, B.G., Beauchamp, M. and Matthews, W.B. (1975) 'Subcortical, somatosensory evoked potentials in man,' *Electroencephalography and Clinical Neurophysiology, 38,* 216.

Taylor, I.G. (1974) 'Deaf children,' *British Journal of Hospital Medicine, 12,* 440.

Chapter 14

Barber, B. and Abbot, W. (1972) *Computing and Operational Research at the London Hospital,* Butterworth, London.

Cordeau, J.P. (1959) 'Monorhythmic frontal delta activity in human electroencephalograms,' *Electroencephalography and Clinical Neurophysiology, 11,* 733.

Krauthammer, W., Last, S.L. Morgan, M.H. and Prior, P.F. (1966) 'EEG Reports – the storage of data in a computer,' *Electroencephalography and Clinical Neurophysiology, 21,* 616.

Rose, S.W., Penry, J.K., White, B.G. and Sato, S. (1973) 'Reliability and validity of visual EEG assessment in third grade children,' *Clinical Electroencephalography, 4,* 197.

Scott, D.F. (1970) *The Psychology of Work,* Duckworth, London.

Volavka, J., Matousek, M., Feldstein, S., Roubicek, J., Prior, P., Scott, D.F., Brezinova, V. and Synek, V. (1973) 'Die Zuverlassigkeit der EEG-Beurteilung' (The reliability of EEG assessment), *Zeitschrift für Elektroenzephalographie Elektromyographie und verwandte Gebiete, 4,* 123.

Chapter 15

Chatrian, G.E., Bergamini, L., Dandey, M., Kloss, D.W., Lennox-Buchthal, M. and Petersen, I. (1974) 'A glossary of terms commonly used by clinical electroencephalographers,' *Electroencephalography and Clinical Neurophysiology, 37,* 538.

Cabral, R. and Scott, D.F. (1975) 'Behaviour therapy in drug resistant epilepsy,' *Proceedings of the Sixth International Symposium on Epilepsy in Brussels in 1973.*

Editorial (1974) 'Internal carotid stenosis,' *British Medical Journal, 1,* 258.

Gazzard, B.J. *et al.* (1974) 'Charcoal haemo-perfusion in the treatment of fulminant hepatic failure,' *Lancet, 1,* 1301.

Geier, S. (1971) 'Minor seizures and behaviour,' *Electroencephalography and Clinical Neurophysiology, 31,* 499.

Goldensohn, E.S., Zablow, W.L. and Stein, B. (1970) 'Inter-relations of form and latency of spike discharge from small areas of the human cortex,' *Electroencephalography and Clinical Neurophysiology, 29,* 321.

Johnson, *et al.* (1975) 'Proceedings of joint meeting of EEG Society and Scandinavian Societies,' *Electroencephalography and Clinical Neurophysiology, 39,* 208.

Kellaway, P. and Petersen, I. (1973) *Automation of Clinical Electroencephalography,* Raven Press, New York.

MacGillivray, B.M. (1974) 'The EEG in epilepsy', Communication delivered at the International League Against Epilepsy, The National Hospital, Queen Square, London, April, 1974.

Maynard, D.E., (1972) 'Separation of sinusoidal components of the human electroencephalogram,' *Nature, 1236,* 228.

Sterman, M.B., MacDonald, L.R. and Stone, R.K. (1974) 'Biofeedback training of the sensory motor electroencephalogram rhythm in man: effects on epilepsy,' *Epilepsia, 15,* 395.

Stevens, J.R., Kodama, H., Lonsbury, B. and Mills L., (1971). 'Ultradian characteristics of spontaneous seizure discharges recorded by radio-telemetry in man,' *Electroencephalography and Clinical Neurophysiology, 31,* 313.

West, L. and Driver, M.V. (1974) 'Antisocial behaviour, barbiturate addiction and associated electroencephalographic changes,' *British Journal of Psychiatry, 125,* 470.

Wolff, H.S., (1967) 'Telemetry of psychophysiological variables,' in *Manual of Psychophysiological Methods,* ed. Venables, P.J. and Martin, I., North Holland, Amsterdam.

Index

G indicates an entry in the Glossary